MW00985891

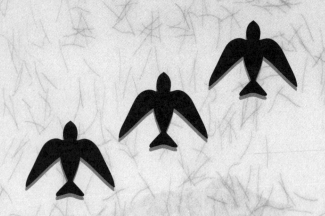

Symptom Management Algorithms
A Handbook for
Palliative Care

Linda Wrede-Seaman, M. D.

Intellicard
P. O. Box 8255,
Yakima, WA 98908

Members of the Palliative Care Resource
Team who have authored significant portions
of this book are:

Dionetta Hudzinski, C.H.R.N.

Ron Jennings, R.Ph.

Matthew Seaman, M.D.

Printed in China

Copyright ©1999 Intellicard, Inc.

Second printing 2002.

Algorithms are used with permission - Providence Yakima Medical Center - Central Washington Service Area

ISBN 1-888411-07-4

Dedication

This book is dedicated to our hospice patients; they have helped to teach us the meaning of life and have inspired us along the way.

Author's special dedication:

To Janet Thielmeyer-Wrede-Umlauf, hospice volunteer, champion of harmonious living, mother and friend.

Refer to website *www.Intelli-card.com* for updates, additions, and revisions to the material in this publication

Table of Contents

Refer to website www.Intelli-card.com for updates, additions, and revisions to the material in this publication

Table of Contents

Table of Contents

Refer to website www.Intelli-card.com for updates, additions,
and revisions to the material in this publication

Table of Contents

Refer to website www.Intelli-card.com for bibliography

Foreward

A commitment to creating a quality life for our dying patients, or any patient requiring palliative care, has led to the development of the enclosed standing orders. Under the supervision of the hospice medical director and referring physician, the algorithmic model provides guidelines that allow pharmacists with prescriptive authority to expedite timely, cost effective relief of pain and other distressing symptoms. Since implementation, the turnaround time for medications to arrive in the homes of our patients has gone from 24-48 hours to an average of 1-2 hours. Patient, caregiver, staff and physician satisfaction have been positively impacted as well as the knowledge base of our home care staff and community physicians.

This booklet reflects the content of Providence Hospice of Yakima's standing orders and serves as an educational tool. These algorithms are useful to professionals working in long term care, home care, outpatient care, or hospital care; they are particularly useful for the fields of palliative medicine, oncology, and hospice care. In many cases, these algorithms can benefit patients in general medicine who are not enrolled in hospice care.

Many steps must be taken to properly implement these algorithms into a cancer center, palliative care center, or hospice program; a summary of these steps is included in the *Overview of the Algorithm Process for Palliative Care*. The author wishes to caution that approval from the state Board of Pharmacy for pharmacists utilizing prescriptive authority must be obtained. It is also recommended that approval from one's hospital pharmacy and therapeutics committee be obtained to streamline care between the hospital and home care setting. For all those utilizing the algorithms, a formal educational in-servicing on the content of the algorithms and the process of communication and documentation is recommended. For further information, please contact the author at Intellicard, PO Box 8255, Yakima, WA 98908. In addition, refer to the Intellicard web site at *www.Intelli-card.com* for supplemental materials, revisions, and a reference list.

Acknowledgments

The author wishes to acknowledge the efforts of the Providence Hospice of Yakima interdisciplinary team in bringing to fruition this dream of creating a more efficient, effective system of caring for the terminally ill. In this revision, special thanks to Ellen Rowley, MSW, Dennis Berthon, MSW, and Ed Cummings, M.Div, who have gently reminded me that physical comfort is incomplete without psychosocial and spiritual comfort. My compliments to the few pharmacists who originally stepped out of their traditional roles, became a part of the homecare team, and stretched into the intimate realm of our dying patients. Special thanks to Mauria Prince, RPh and Dionetta Hudzinski, CHRN who took the ideas, put them on paper, and created the initial version of these algorithms. Thanks also to the other important supporters: Glenda Abercrombie, RN (former hospice manager) and Wanda Lennon, RN (program administrator). Lastly, special thanks for the encouragement received from the American Academy of Hospice and Palliative Medicine. This organization provided the training and foundation to this fledgling medical director who wanted to make a difference; the Academy continues to foster the vision of *"a good death"* for all individuals around the world.

Overview of the Algorithm Process for Palliative Care

The goal of the algorithms is to deliver consistent, timely care to our terminal patients. As symptoms arise, they are treated based on thorough medical assessments and physician approved algorithms. This uniform approach to managed care assists in containing costs and creates a standard of care in the community.

The symptom management algorithms allow for a team approach involving the referring physician, medical director, nurse, pharmacist, volunteer coordinator, billing representative, social worker, chaplain, nurses's aide, program administrator, patient and family caregivers. As each patient is admitted to the hospice program, the interdisciplinary team meets to discuss the patient assessment and create a plan of care. The algorithms are instituted when orders are signed by the referring physician and the program medical director. In developing these algorithms, an effort was made to allow for flexibility that is required for individual patient differences and to accommodate physician preferences for various therapies and medications. The medical director may then act in concert with the attending physician to expedite care. It is the medical director's obligation to oversee the proper development and implementation of the algorithms.

Pharmacists on the staff of Providence Yakima Medical Center have prescriptive authority granted by the Washington State Board of Pharmacy. With this authority and the signed orders of the program medical director and attending physician, the pharmacists can write prescriptions and dispense medications necessary for treatment. This process facilitates timely administration of needed medications. By policy, any action taken within the algorithm, particularly medications dispensed, must be reported to the patient's physician within 24 hours. In addition, documentation of the outcome of the therapeutic action is also required to ensure quality of care.

The symptom management algorithms have helped standardize hospice and palliative medicine, home care, and institutional care. Working together, end of life care can be comfortable, dignified and an opportunity to celebrate any individual's life story.

Symptom Management Algorithm Process

Patient admitted to program

↓

Assessment/information gathering
Patient meets hospice criteria

↓

Interdisciplinary plan of care developed

↓

Communication with referring physician

↓

Approval given to begin algorithms
Medical Director signs admission orders
Algorithms instituted as symptoms arise

↓

Ongoing assessment and evaluation

↓

Current algorithm step not working...
Start next step

↔

Pharmacist writes prescription and notifies physician within 24 hours

Nurse/Pharmacist consult
Physician as needed

↓

Protocol completed

↓

Physician/Nurse/Pharmacist coordinate further care plans
Medical Director consulted as needed

↓

Pharmacist calls Physician for further orders and communicates information to Nurse

Agitation Assessment

Assessment guidelines:

- Assess pain level - differentiate acute exacerbation of chronic pain versus acute onset of new pain (See *Pain Algorithms*)
- Assess sleep deprivation? (See *Sleep Disorder Algorithm*)
- Assess medications based upon the patient's ability to take oral medications and current weight (assess for weight loss)
- Anxiety producing medications (*i.e. corticosteroids*) present?
- Is patient withdrawing from opioids or barbiturates?
- Paradoxical effects of certain medications especially in geriatric population?
- Document history of tobacco, alcohol, or other substance abuse. Is there recent abstinence precipitating withdrawal?
- Document stage of disease state and functional status (See *Appendix*)
- Document a *Quality of Life Score* (See *Appendix*)
- Document the *FAST* score (See *Appendix*)
- Metabolic state - i.e., electrolyte disturbance, hypoxia present? (See *Dyspnea Algorithm*)
- Expression of psychiatric disturbance? If depressed, see *Depression Algorithm*. Perform mini-mental status examination (See *MMSE in Appendix*)
- Unexplained - impending catastrophic event?
- Fecal impaction - or urinary retention? (See *Bowel Treatment Stepped Care Program* and *Bladder Algorithm*)
- Respiratory distress? (See *Dyspnea Algorithm*)
- Is there unfinished business? Are there unmet spiritual needs? Consult Chaplain (See *Psychosocial* and *Spiritual Assessment/Intervention Guides*)
- Is this terminal agitation? (See *Terminal Agitation Algorithm*)

Physician-Nurse-Pharmacist consultation for any etiology not addressed in algorithm

Implement appropriate non-pharmacologic interventions

Initiate *Agitation Algorithm* and/or proceed to other associated algorithms

Non-Pharmacologic Interventions

• Active, empathic listening • Simplified, subdued environment and reduce distractions and noise • Well lit surroundings with familiar objects and familiar faces • Conversation with the patient and family should be calm and reassuring • Create structured, predictable routines • Assess spiritual needs and intervene as needed • Allow time for patient to talk freely about his/her concerns • Assess socialization needs of patient • Relaxation/visualization/distraction therapy • Aromatherapy • Therapeutic touch • Massage therapy • Pet therapy • Offer relaxation tapes • Patient and family education regarding treatment options, medications and anticipated effects

Agitation Treatment Algorithm

- Lorazepam[†] 1.0 - 2.0 mg Q 4 hours PRN; PO/SL/PR/IM/IV/SC (See *Anxiety Algorithm* for titration parameters)
- Haloperidol*[†] 5.0 mg PO/IM/IV/SC.

  Titrate up by 0.5 mg Q 4 h until desired effect achieved (MDD 20 mg)
- Trazadone[†] 50 mg PO Q HS (MDD 300 mg)
- Consider therapy for alcohol or nicotine withdrawal when the history and physical exam suggest a withdrawal syndrome. Physician - Nurse - Pharmacist consultation to discuss use of nicotine patch or alcohol withdrawal protocol
- For sleep disturbance, see *Sleep Disorder Algorithm*
- For anxiety, see *Anxiety Algorithm*

  [†] Use half the listed dose in elderly or debilitated patients

No Relief

- Consider psychiatric evaluation. Document MMSE (Mini Mental Status Examiniation - see *Appendix*; see also *Psychosocial and Spiritual Algorithms*).
- For patients with psychosis, especially schizophrenia with a significant anger component, consider trial of resperidol 0.5 mg PO BID; may double the dose QD based on the clinical response. MDD 6 mg. Alternatively, for aggressive patients, divalproex 125 mg PO BID. Reassess for efficacy in 7 days; monitor side effects.
- For patients with an obsessive compulsive disorder, consider trial of fluvoxamine (Luvox) 50 mg PO HS (starting dose) and increase by 50 mg increments every 4 - 7 days (MDD 300 mg) Reassess for efficacy in 7 days; monitor side effects.
- For patients with depression, see *Depression Algorithm*.

No Relief

Physician - Nurse - Pharmacist consultation for further orders. Consider continuous infusion of haloperidol (SC or IV).

See *Terminal Agitation Algorithm*. Consider alternative antipsychotic medication.

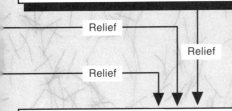

Acute and severe agitation

For acute and severe agitation:

• Lorazepam 2 mg / haloperidol 5 mg (intramuscular combination)

Use half the dose for geriatric or debilitated patients. Repeat in 15 - 30 minutes if needed. Monitor blood pressure and pulse. Continue therapy as needed for 48 - 72 hours, then reassess need to maintain therapy.

For acute agitation with significant anger component:

• Divalproex (Depakene) 150 mg PO BID. Reassess efficacy in 7 days.

Relief

Relief

Relief

Evaluate regularly. If possible, attempt to discontinue pharmacologic therapy. When switching from an antipsychotic agent where a partial response has been observed, taper the medication while initiating therapy with a new medication.

*Avoid butyrophenones in patients with Parkinson's disease. Watch for extrapyramidal symptoms.

Anxiety Assessment

Assessment guidelines:
- Assess pain level - differentiate acute exacerbation of chronic pain versus acute onset of new pain (*See Pain Algorithms*)
- Document stage of disease state and functional status (See *Appendix*)
- Assess sleep deprivation? (See *Sleep Disorder Algorithm*)
- Anxiety producing medications (*i.e. corticosteroids*) or withdrawal of opiates or barbiturates?
- Paradoxical effects of certain medications especially in geriatric population?
- Assess medications based upon the patient's ability to take oral medications and based upon current weight (assess for weight loss)
- Document history of tobacco, alcohol, or other substance abuse. Is there recent abstinence or evidence of withdrawal?
- Document a *Quality of Life Score* (See *Appendix*)
- Document the *FAST* score (See *Appendix*)
- Metabolic state - i.e., electrolyte disturbance; hypoxia (See *Dyspnea Algorithm*)
- Psychiatric disturbance or depression? Perform mini-mental status examination (See *MMSE* in *Appendix;* see *Psychosocial Assessment/Intervention Guide* and *Depression Algorithm*)
- Unexplained - impending catastrophic event?
- Fecal impaction - or urinary retention? (See *Bowel Treatment Stepped Care Program and Bladder Algorithm*)
- Respiratory distress? (See *Dyspnea Algorithm*)
- Unmet spiritual needs? Unfinished business? Consult Chaplain (See *Psychosocial and Spiritual Assessment/Intervention Guide*)
- Is this terminal agitation? (See *Terminal Agitation Algorithm*)

Physician-Nurse-Pharmacist consultation for any etiology not addressed in algorithm

Implement appropriate non-pharmacologic interventions

Initiate *Anxiety Algorithm* and/or proceed to other associated algorithms

Non-Pharmacologic Interventions

- Active, empathic listening • Subdued environment/reduce stimulus • Softly lighted surroundings with familiar objects and familiar faces • Conversation with the patient and family should be calm and reassuring • Allow time for patient to talk freely about his/her concerns • Aromatherapy • Relaxation/visualization/distraction therapy • Offer relaxation tapes • Massage therapy • Therapeutic touch • Create simple predictable routines • Pet therapy • Patient and family education regarding treatment options, medications and anticipated effects

Anxiety Treatment Algorithm

Lorazepam 0.5 mg Q 4 h PRN; PO/SL/PR/IM/IV/SC

Relief → Continue lorazepam 0.5 mg Q 4 h PRN PO/IM/SL/IV/PR/SC

Relief → Continue lorazepam or diazepam at effective dose; evaluate regularly in effort to taper or discontinue. Consider buspirone (Buspar) 10 mg PO TID (MDD 60 mg)

No Relief after 24 hours → Lorazepam - Increase to 1 mg Q 4 h PRN. If not adequate, titrate up by 0.5 mg - 2 mg Q 4 h PRN until desired effect achieved; MDD 12 mg. Alternatively, diazepam 2.5 - 5 mg PO/IM/IV/PR Q 8 h - if not adequate, titrate up by 2 - 5 mg Q 4 h until desired effect achieved; MDD 40 mg

No Relief ↓

- Haloperidol* 1.0 - 2.0 mg PO/IM/IV/SC Q 4 hours

Haloperidol - titrate up by 0.5 mg Q 4 h as needed; MDD 20 mg

Relief → Continue haloperidol; evaluate regularly in effort to taper or discontinue

No Relief → Titrate dose of haloperidol up until desired effect achieved*

No relief after 24 hours - Physician - Nurse - Pharmacist consultation for further orders (See *Agitation Algorithm* or *Terminal Agitation Algorithm*; See *Adjuvant Medication Guide*)

* Avoid butyrophenones in patients with Parkinson's disease. Watch for extrapyramidal side effects.

Appetite Loss Assessment

Assessment Guidelines:
- How long has appetite been suppressed? Sudden or progressive?
- Has there been significant weight loss? Over what time frame?
- Is there a distortion of smells / tastes?
- Does patient have AIDS?
- Is dysphagia present?
- Document stage of disease and function status (See *Appendix*)
- Assess medications based upon the patient's ability to take oral medications and based upon current weight
- Document a *Quality of Life Score* (See *Appendix*)
- Document the *FAST* score (See *Appendix*)
- Assess oral cavity - mucous membranes, teeth, gingiva, lips (See *Oral Candidiasis or Mucositis Treatment Algorithm* if indicated)
- Assess for depression; would pt benefit from therapy? (See *Depression or Anxiety Treatment Algorithm*)
- Review other medications; is patient already on steroids?
- Assess nausea and bowel function. Is patient constipated?
- Discuss patient directive regarding nutrition and hydration.
- Assess nutritional status (documentation of albumin, protein)

Physician - Nurse - Pharmacist consultation for any etiology not addressed in algorithm

If distressing to family and patient, implement appropriate non - pharmacologic interventions

If distressing to family and patient initiate, *Appetite Loss Algorithm* and / or proceed to other associated algorithms

Non-Pharmacologic Interventions

- Educate patient and family regarding treatment options, benefits and anticipated effects • Allay family fears / anxiety regarding the patient "starving" • Initiate nutritional counseling if desired • Provide high caloric liquid preparations • Consider prepared meals
- Encourage patient to partake of small portions of highly enjoyable foods with their family meals • Aromatherapy • Therapeutic touch
- Mouth care, ice chips, cold beverages as oral intake declines

Appetite Loss Treatment Algorithm

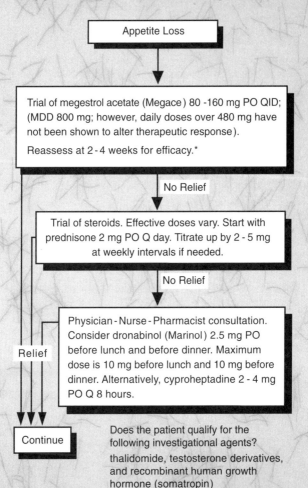

Appetite Loss

Trial of megestrol acetate (Megace) 80 -160 mg PO QID; (MDD 800 mg; however, daily doses over 480 mg have not been shown to alter therapeutic response).

Reassess at 2 - 4 weeks for efficacy.*

No Relief

Trial of steroids. Effective doses vary. Start with prednisone 2 mg PO Q day. Titrate up by 2 - 5 mg at weekly intervals if needed.

No Relief

Physician - Nurse - Pharmacist consultation. Consider dronabinol (Marinol) 2.5 mg PO before lunch and before dinner. Maximum dose is 10 mg before lunch and 10 mg before dinner. Alternatively, cyproheptadine 2 - 4 mg PO Q 8 hours.

Relief

Continue

Does the patient qualify for the following investigational agents?

thalidomide, testosterone derivatives, and recombinant human growth hormone (somatropin)

*Document weight every 2 weeks. If no response, discontinue or taper therapy after 4 - 8 weeks.

Ascites Assessment

Assessment Guidelines:
- Document stage of disease and functional status (See *Appendix*)
- Assess medications based upon the patient's ability to take oral medications and based upon current weight (assess for weight loss)
- Assess patient's nutritional status (document protein, albumin)
- Document the *Quality of Life Score* (See *Appendix*)
- Document the *FAST* score (See *Appendix*)
- Presence of pain or discomfort (*See Pain Algorithm*)
- Respiratory status? (*See Dyspnea Algorithm*)
- Review diet and meds for contributing cause
- Substance abuse history?
- HIV status; AIDS?
- History of hepatic/renal disease? Coagulopathy?
- History of cardiac disease?
- Presence of metastatic disease?
- Measure abdominal girth; weigh patient if possible
- Assess for extent of peripheral edema
- Discuss possible indications for paracentesis; document patient's preferences

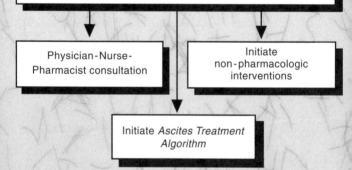

Physician-Nurse-Pharmacist consultation

Initiate non-pharmacologic interventions

Initiate *Ascites Treatment Algorithm*

Non-Pharmacologic Interventions

- Educate patient and family regarding etiology, treatment options, medications, and anticipated effects • Bedrest • Hospital bed
- Patient will usually be more comfortable sitting up in chair with legs elevated or in bed with head of bed elevated and legs slightly elevated • Good skin care and hygiene are essential • Frequent mouth care if fluid restriction is necessary • Renal Preservation Diet/Sodium/Fluid restricted diet (See *Appendix*)

Ascites Treatment Algorithm

Restrict sodium intake and fluids. Consider dietician consultation (See *Appendix for Renal Preservation or sodium restricted diet*)

↓

Patient will be more comfortable sitting up; elevate head of bed with legs slightly elevated

Start diuretics: spironolactone (start at 50 mg QD). If not effective after 5 days, increase to 100 mg PO QD; reassess frequently and titrate as necessary. If liver failure is present, start lactulose 30 - 45 mL Q 6 hours; titrate dose to promote soft stools

↓

Good skin care and oral hygiene

No Relief

Ascites should be reduced only to the extent necessary to relieve patient's symptoms of dyspnea and / or discomfort

Continue

↓

Physician - Nurse - Pharmacist consultation to consider paracentesis for comfort if above interventions are not effective

Bladder Assessment

Assessment Guidelines
- Document stage of disease and functional status (See *Appendix*)
- Assess medications based upon the patient's ability to take oral medications and based upon current weight (assess for weight loss)
- Document the *Quality of Life Score* (See *Appendix*)
- Document the *FAST* score (See *Appendix*)
- Assess oral fluid intake
- UTI symptoms? (See *Bladder Spasm Algorithm*)
- Fecal impaction? (See *Bowel Treatment Stepped Care Program*)
- CNS dysfunction? (*confused, sedated, comatose*) (See *Appendix* for Mini Mental Status Exam)
- Spinal cord compression? (See *Adjuvant Medication Guide* in *Appendix* for high dose steroid therapy)
- Urinary retention with or without overflow?
- Attempt to quantitate if urine output $\geq$ 2 cc/kg/hr (If anuric, see *Anuria Assessment Algorithm*)
- Are medication side effects contributing to symptoms?
- Are opioids contributing to urinary retention? (See *Appendix* for *Adjuvant Medication Guide*)

Physician-Nurse-Pharmacist consultation

Initiate *Anuria Algorithm, Bladder Spasm Algorithm* or *Urinary Incontinence Algorithm* and/or proceed to other associated algorithms

Implement appropriate non-pharmacologic interventions

Non-Pharmacologic Interventions

- Educate patient and family on treatment options, medications and anticipated effects • If possible, treat the underlying cause of incontinence • Consider use of incontinence pads • Maintain good skin care to prevent skin breakdown • See *Skin Care Algorithm*
- Teach family or caregivers how to care for incontinent or catheterized patient • Consider the use of external catheter in males • Aromatherapy • Cotton ball soaked in peppermint tincture in bed pan

Urinary Incontinence Algorithm

See *Bladder Assessment* and *Skin Care Guidelines* prior to initiating. Catheterize for post void residual; use lidocaine 2% gel.

- For new onset incontinence, urge incontinence or dysuria, send urinalysis. See *Bladder Spasm Algorithm* for guidelines on suspected urinary tract infections.
- Consider Pyridium (phenazopyridine) 100 - 200 mg PO TID for transient dysuria. Educate patient / caregiver on darkening of urine.

| Over 50 mL | Less than 50 mL |

- Assess patient/caregiver tolerance regarding the use of incontinence pads; if tolerated, begin pads.
- Is skin breakdown a problem? (See *Skin Care Guidelines*)

Leave catheter in place. If there is urge incontinence or bladder spasm, see *Bladder Spasm Algorithm*. For catheter options, see *Skin Care Guidelines - Incontinence*

Have symptoms resolved?

No　　　Yes

Continue. Frequently reassess the skin. Reassess patient and caregiver tolerance.

If catheter becomes plugged, irrigate with normal saline PRN. Is the patient a candidate for self catheterization or external catheter?

Insert retention catheter. Use lidocaine 2% gel.

Change catheter every month and as needed

Anuria Algorithm

- See *Bladder Assessment*
- See *Renal Preservation Diet* in *Appendix* if indicated.
- See *Ascites Algorithm* if indicated.

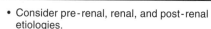

No urine output in over
8 hours

- Consider pre-renal, renal, and post-renal etiologies.
- Assess intake of fluids in past 24 hours. Are there signs and symptoms of dehydration?
- Document stage of disease and functional status (See *Appendix*)
- Is there known renal insufficiency?
- Assess for pelvic involvement of disease process?
- Assess level of consciousness of patient
- Assess caregiver reliability
- What is the patient's directive on intravenous hydration?

Insert retention catheter if appropriate
(use 2% lidocaine gel)

Skin problems related to incontinence: Consider adult incontinence pads or external catheter as alternative to retention catheter; implement skin care interventions
(See *Skin Care Algorithm*)

Bladder Spasms Assessment

Assessment guidelines:
- UTI symptoms?
- Fluid intake - adequate for stage of disease?
- Assess diet for offending foods and spices
- For indwelling catheter - assess function, catheter size, and balloon - (too large?)
- Assess for tumor encroachment upon bladder or urethra (*Physician-Nurse-Pharmacist consultation*)
- Assess for neurologic problems, stroke, cord lesions, or multiple sclerosis contributing to detrusor instability (*Physician–Nurse consultation*)
- Assess for past history of radiation to pelvic area?
- Document stage of disease and functional status (See *Appendix*)
- Assess for blood in urine (*Physician-Nurse-Pharmacist consultation*)

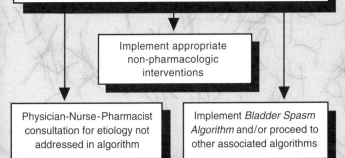

Implement appropriate non-pharmacologic interventions

Physician-Nurse-Pharmacist consultation for etiology not addressed in algorithm

Implement *Bladder Spasm Algorithm* and/or proceed to other associated algorithms

Non-Pharmacologic Interventions

- Patient and family education for treatment options • Adjust fluid intake (cut fluids back; in some cases increasing fluids may stretch the bladder and decrease spasms) • Biofeedback • Relaxation techniques • Imagery • Hypnosis • Aromatherapy • Sit or stand to void • Encouragement • Timed voidings • Remove foley catheter for a trial period • Consider dietician consultation • In some patients, frequent self catheterization may be an option

Bladder Spasms Treatment

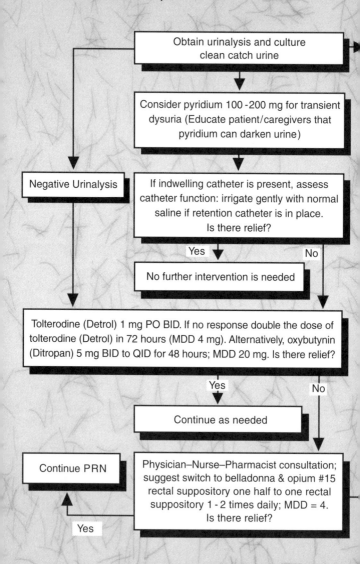

Obtain urinalysis and culture
clean catch urine

Consider pyridium 100 - 200 mg for transient
dysuria (Educate patient/caregivers that
pyridium can darken urine)

Negative Urinalysis

If indwelling catheter is present, assess
catheter function: irrigate gently with normal
saline if retention catheter is in place.
Is there relief?

Yes   No

No further intervention is needed

Tolterodine (Detrol) 1 mg PO BID. If no response double the dose of
tolterodine (Detrol) in 72 hours (MDD 4 mg). Alternatively, oxybutynin
(Ditropan) 5 mg BID to QID for 48 hours; MDD 20 mg. Is there relief?

Yes   No

Continue as needed

Continue PRN

Physician–Nurse–Pharmacist consultation;
suggest switch to belladonna & opium #15
rectal suppository one half to one rectal
suppository 1 - 2 times daily; MDD = 4.
Is there relief?

Yes

Positive Urinalysis

↓

Start empiric antibiotics. Consider prior urine culture and sensitivity results and drug allergies.

Empiric drugs include:

- trimethoprim and sulfamethoxazole (1 DS PO BID) for 3 days
- cephalexin (500 mg PO QID) for ten days
- ciprofloxacin (500 mg PO BID) for ten days

↓

Obtain catheterized urine C & S if the infection fails to improve with empiric therapy

↓

For chronic and recurrent infections, consider suppressive therapy with nitrofurantoin macrocrystals (Macrobid) 50 - 100 mg PO daily.

↓ Continued symptoms

Physician − Nurse − Pharmacist consultation

↑

No

Bowel Assessment

Assessment:
- Is patient on opioids? For adjustment of opioid dosing, see *Pain Management Guidelines*
- Are other mediations affecting bowel function?
- Bowel sounds - present - hypo/hyperactive?
- Palpate for abdominal tenderness or presence of mass
- Check for fecal impaction
- Assess usual pattern of bowel movements
- Date of last bowel movement?
- What interventions have been tried?
- Presence of nausea/vomiting? (See *Nausea Algorithm*)
- Assess fluid intake and dietary intake?
- Is patient neutropenic or thrombocytopenic?
- Document stage of disease and functional status (See *Appendix*)
- Is there suspected partial or complete bowel obstruction?

Implement non-pharmacologic interventions

Physician-Nurse-Pharmacist consultation for etiology not addressed in algorithm; consult if patient is neutropenic or thrombocytopenic

Implement *Bowel Treatment Stepped Care Program* if constipated, impacted, on opioid therapy, or other drugs which might contribute to constipation. For loose stools, see *Diarrhea Algorithm*.

Non-Pharmacologic Interventions

- Increase dietary fiber (fruits, fruit paste*, vegetables, salads)
- Encourage increased mobility including passive or active range of motion exercises if possible
- Increase oral fluid intake
- Consider one cup of stimulant such as caffeine in the morning
- If nauseated, see *Nausea Non-Pharmacologic Interventions* (*Yakima Fruit Paste recipe in Appendix*)

Bowel Treatment - Stepped Care Program

Step 1 - Begin with a stool softener and laxative. Use one of the following choices:

- Docusate Sodium 250 mg daily to BID (*rarely used alone*)
- Fruit paste* 1-2 tablespoonfuls daily
- Docusate Sodium 100 mg/casanthranol 30 mg (*Doxidan*); 1 cap TID (*range: 1-2 capsules QD to TID*)
- Docusate Sodium 50 mg plus Sennosides 8.6 mg (*Senokot-S*); 1 tablet TID (*range: 1-4 tabs QD to TID; also, guide dosing as follows: 1 tab/4 mg hydromorphone, 1 tab/15 mg morphine*)

Step 2 - If no bowel movement in any 48 hour period, add one of the following:

- Senna (*Senokot*) 2-3 tablets PO QD
- Bisacodyl (*Dulcolax*) 10-15 mg PO QD (*range: 5 mg to 15 mg PO QD*)
- Milk of magnesia 30-60 mL PO QD (*range: QD to BID*)
- Lactulose (*Chronulac 10 gm/15 mL*) 30-45 mL QD (*range: 15-60 mL QD; larger doses are usually divided BID-TID*)

Step 3 - **If no bowel movement by 72 hours, perform rectal examination to rule out impaction; try one of the following:

- Bisacodyl (*Dulcolax*) 10 mg RS
- Magnesium citrate 8 oz PO
- Mineral oil 30-60 ml PO
- Fleet enema or warm saline enema

Step 4 - **If rectal stool impacted try the following:

- Manually disimpact if stool is soft enough (*consider pretreatment of patient with analgesic or sedative*)
- Soften with glycerin suppository, mineral oil or olive oil retention enema, then disimpact manually
- Follow up with enema(s) of choice (*tap water or soap suds enema*) until clear and then increase intensity of daily bowel program
- If rectal pain or discomfort suggest hemorrhoidal ointment or suppositories with warm sitz baths. (*Preparation H, Anusol HC, Benzocaine [Hurricaine] Suppositories etc.*) Also, consider use of rectal wipes (Tucks)

* Yakima Fruit Paste recipe in Appendix

** Do not implement step C or D in neutropenic/thrombocytopenic patient before physician-nurse consultation

Candidiasis–Oral Assessment

Assessment Guidelines:
- Dysphagia without observable signs of candidiasis
- Assess oral cavity (*including tongue, gingiva, mucous membranes, lips and saliva*)
- Assess voice quality and swallowing ability
- Assess for presence of creamy white curd-like patches in oral cavity
- Assess oral hygiene practices
- Assess oral intake
- Assess use of steroid inhalers
- AIDS?
- Assess current medications for the possibility of drug induced oral mucositis that may resemble candidiasis (i.e. recent sulfa therapy)
- Is patient at risk for graft versus host disease? (i.e previous bone marrow transplant)

Initiate *Candidiasis - Oral Treatment Algorithm*

Physician-Nurse-Pharmacist consultation for etiology not addressed in this algorithm

Implement appropriate non-pharmacologic interventions

Non-Pharmacologic Interventions

• Educate patient and family regarding treatment options, medications and anticipated effects • Warm salt water rinses (swish, gargle) • Brush tongue as well as teeth with soft tooth brush • Rinse mouth with nonalcoholic mouth wash (glyoxide peroxide or cetyl pyridium in glycerin) Q 2 hours while awake • Soft diet for severe dysphagia • Rinse mouth with dilute hydrogen peroxide

Candidiasis–Oral Treatment Algorithm

- Nystatin suspension 5 mL (500,000 U) swish and swallow QID; hold in mouth 2 - 5 minutes
- For associated oral pain, see *Mucositis Algorithm*

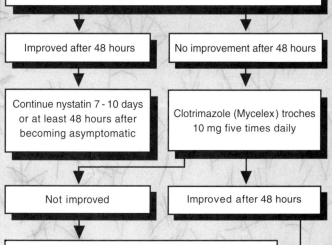

Improved after 48 hours	No improvement after 48 hours
Continue nystatin 7 - 10 days or at least 48 hours after becoming asymptomatic	Clotrimazole (Mycelex) troches 10 mg five times daily
Not improved	Improved after 48 hours

Trial of oral antifungal: fluconazole (Diflucan) 200 mg loading dose then 100 mg QD for 5 - 7 days. Titrate dose up as needed. Daily doses in excess of 400 mg are not recommended. Alternatively, consider therapy with itraconazole (Sporanox) 200 mg PO QD for 14 days. For refractory cases, consider amphotericin B solution (0.1 mg/mL) 15 mL QID swish and spit.

Physician–Nurse–Pharmacist consultation. Explore the possibility of a medication reaction (i.e. sulfa reaction) and graft versus host disease (when the medical history suggests this possibility).

Continue clotrimazole (Mycelex) troches 10 mg five times daily for 14 days

Candidiasis–Perineal Assessment

Assessment Guidelines:
- Document stage of disease and functional status (See *Appendix*)
- Recent antibiotic therapy?
- Recent chemotherapy or radiation treatments?
- Perineal discharge present? (color, odor, consistency)
- Assess for perineal lesions and/or rash
- Pruritus and/or pain? (See *Pruritus and/or Pain Algorithm*)
- Dysuria - (See *Bladder Algorithms*)
- Assess personal hygiene practices
- AIDS?
- In a female patient, assess for vaginitis
- Assess for diarrhea

Initiate *Candidiasis-Perineal Treatment Algorithm* and/or proceed to other associated algorithms

Physician-Nurse-Pharmacist consultation for etiology not addressed in this algorithm

Implement appropriate non-pharmacologic interventions (See *Skin Care Guidelines*)

Non-Pharmacologic Interventions

•Educate patient and family regarding treatment options, medications and anticipated effects •Apply powder or dry padding in potential problem areas of patients to prevent irritation and Candida growth •Check high risk patients frequently (obese, diabetics, chronic antibiotic or steroid therapy) •Cleanse 3-4 times per day minimum, especially after defecation or urination. •Air dry involved area for brief times throughout the day

Candidiasis–Perineal Treatment Algorithm

Clotrimazole 1% cream (Gynelotrimin) applied BID*.
For intravaginal source of candidiasis, apply clotrimazole 1%
cream intravaginally BID as well. If diarrhea is present, see
Diarrhea Assessment and Treatment Algorithms.

Improved after 48 hours

No improvement after
48 hours

Terconazole 0.4% cream apply Q HS. For intravaginal
source of candidiasis, apply terconazole 0.4% cream
intravaginally QD as well

Continue clotrimazole
7 - 14 days

Improved after 48 hours

Not improved

Continue for 7 days

Physician–Nurse–Pharmacist consultation; Consider ketoconazole
2% cream (Nizoral) QD–BID for two weeks and fluconazole
(Diflucan) one time dose of 150 mg PO. Alternatively,
itraconazole (Sporanox) 200 mg daily for 7 - 10 days (use with
caution due to multiple drug interactions)

* This product is available over-the-counter along with
miconazole (Monistat)

Cough Assessment

Assessment Guidelines:
- Assess stage of disease (*ECOG scale*); is hemoptysis present suggesting tumor invasion?
- Is the patient dyspneic? (See *Dyspnea Algorithm*)
- Does the patient have cardiac or pulmonary disease?
- Assess for frequency and duration of cough
- Assess for associated fever, chills, myalgias?
- Is there sputum production? If so, what is the color of the sputum?
- Assess for pulmonary edema, presence of rales, hepatomegaly, pleural effusion, or ascites
  (See *Dyspnea Algorithm* and *Ascites Algorithm*)
- Review medications; is the patient on ACE inhibitors?
- Are oral secretions contributing to cough?
  (See *Secretions Algorithm*)
- Assess patient's hydration status
- Does the patient smoke?
- Is there a wood burning source of heat?
- Assess for allergic conditions. Are there signs and symptoms of sinus trouble?
- Does the patient have symptoms of gastroesophageal reflux?
  (See *Gastroesophageal Reflux Algorithm*)
- Assess oxygenation. Record pulse oximetry. Are there indications for supplemental oxygen?

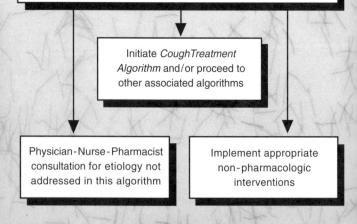

Initiate *CoughTreatment Algorithm* and/or proceed to other associated algorithms

Physician-Nurse-Pharmacist consultation for etiology not addressed in this algorithm

Implement appropriate non-pharmacologic interventions

Non-Pharmacologic Interventions

• Educate patient and family regarding treatment options, medications and anticipated effects • Humidify the room • Elevate head of bed • Throat lozenges • Frequent sips of water • Eliminate allergens in the environment if possible

Cough Treatment Algorithm

Cough[1]

Signs/symptoms of infection

Signs/symptoms of broncho-spasm (mainly allergic symptoms)

If symptoms suggest bronchitis or pneumonia, begin empiric antibiotics consider drug allergies, drug interactions and clinical circumstances:
- Zithromax 500 mg PO day one, then 250 mg PO daily on day 2-5
- Levaquin 500 mg PO daily for ten days
- Biaxin 500 mg PO BID for ten days
- Amoxicillin 250-500 mg PO TID for ten days
- Bactrim DS one PO BID for ten days

Inhaled beta-agonists:
- Metaproterenol (Alupent) - 2 inhalations Q 4-6 h
- Albuterol (Proventil) - 2 inhalations Q 4-6 h
  Does bronchospasm continue?

Yes

Consider adding
- Triamcinalone inhalation (Azmacort) two inhalations QID
- Ipratropium bromide (Atrovent) 1-2 inhalations QID
  Does bronchospasm continue?

Yes

- Prednisone - 40 mg PO daily for two days, followed by tapering the dose by 50% each day (total course of prednisone is seven days)
  Does bronchospasm continue?

Yes

If symptoms continue or worsen despite therapy, Physician-Nurse-Pharmacist consultation

If improved, complete therapy and reassess.

Signs/symptoms of
pulmonary edema

See *Dyspnea Treatment
Algorithm*

Cough is disturbing to
patient or family[1]

- Dextromethorphan (Delsym) 10 - 20 mg PO Q 4 hrs
- Guaifenesin and codeine syrup (Robitussin AC) - 10 mL PO Q 4 hours
- Benzonatate (Tessalon Perles) one PO TID
  Improved?

Yes

No

- Hydrocodone and chlorpheniramine polistirex extended release syrup (Tussionex) - 5 mL PO BID
- Hydrocodone and guaifenesin syrup (Vicodin Tuss) 5 - 10 mL PO Q 4 hours PRN
  Improved?

Yes

No

Nebulized local anesthetics.[2] For refractory cough, give patient a sip of water. Then administer nebulized 0.25% - 0.5% bupivacaine 5 mL Q 4 hours PRN (Maximum recommended dose 30 mL/day). Alternatively, lidocaine 1% 2.5 mL Q 4 hours PRN.
Improved?

Yes

No

If symptoms continue or worsen despite therapy, Physician - Nurse - Pharmacist consultation

If symptoms improve, continue therapy. As signs and symptoms improve, attempt to wean therapy

---

[1] For thick secretions, try nebulized normal saline 5 mL Q 4 hrs PRN. Also, try potassium iodide expectorant (PIMA) 5 mL - 10 mL PO TID PRN.

[2] Since these agents decrease the gag reflex, there is a slight risk of aspiration; this should be discussed with the patient and caregivers. The patient should be NPO for 1 hour pre and post treatment.

Cultural Sensitivity Guidelines

General Questions to ask

- How do you describe the problem? What do you think has caused your illness?
- We all have favorite family remedies that we use when our loved ones are sick. What have you or your family done so far to treat this problem?
- Do you know of anyone else that can help you with this problem? (family, healers, others)
- Have you seen anyone else to get help with this problem? If so, what did they say was wrong and what did they recommend? Have you tried it?
- What else can I (or our team) do to help you?

Quick self-check for cross-cultural medical care

- Understand your own cultural values and biases.
- Acquire basic knowledge of cultural values, health beliefs and nutrition practices for patient groups routinely served.
- Be respectful of, interested in and understanding of other cultures without being judgmental.

Enhancing communication (See *Psychosocial Assessment*)

- Determine the level of fluency in English and arrange for an interpreter if needed.
- Ask how the patient prefers to be addressed.
- Allow the patient to choose seating for comfortable personal space and eye contact.
- Avoid body language that may be offensive or misunderstood.
- Speak directly to the patient, whether or not an interpreter is present.
- Choose a speech rate and style that promotes understanding and demonstrates respect for the client.
- Avoid slang, technical words, and complex sentences.
- Use open-ended questions or questions phrased in several ways to obtain information.
- Determine the patient's reading ability before using written materials; translate or use an interpreter if necessary.

Promoting positive change

- Build on cultural practices. Reinforce those which are positive. Promote change only in those which are harmful.
- Check for patient and family understanding and acceptance of recommendations.
- Remember that not all seeds of knowledge fall into a fertile environment to produce change; of those that do, some will take years to germinate.
- Be patient. Provide counseling in a culturally appropriate environment to promote positive health behavior

Cultural Sensitivity Guidelines

In reality it is not possible to stereotype individuals or cultural groups; with this in mind, a few general points will be listed regarding selected cultures:

Hispanic (Mexican Americans)

- Determine primary and secondary languages.
- There is great diversity in education levels. Determine reading skills and, when necessary, provide good verbal/visual instruction and demonstration.
- Silence sometimes indicates a lack of agreement or understanding with the plan of care.
- In general, handshaking is considered appropriate but wait for permission for closer touch.
- In greeting, it is respectful to address formally, especially with elders and married women.
- When dealing with a serious or terminal illness, the family may be reluctant to share knowledge of prognosis with the ill family member, believing concern and worry will worsen health status.
- The family structure is usually nuclear with extended family and godparents (compadres).
- Traditionally the father or oldest male is head of household and holds the ultimate decision-making authority.
- Mothers publicly defer to their husbands but hold great authority in the family - particularly with children.
- Support systems for help with care are usually first sought within immediate and extended family. Extended families are obligated to attend to the dying and pay their respects; pregnant women are often prohibited from direct care or attending funerals.
- Women are expected to be the primary caregivers. In some cases, if a family member has an open wound, care may not be given for fear of "catching" the illness.
- Self-care frequently involves self-medication and use of traditional resources. A *curandero* is a general practitioner of Mexican folk healing. *Yerbalistas* are herbalists. *Soradoras* are massage therapists.
- Diet may also play an important part in Hispanic symptom management; a traditional belief is that the four bodily *humors* (blood, phlegm, yellow bile, black bile) must be kept in balance.
- Spiritual amulets, medallions or rosary beads are expected to be near the patient.
- Religious rites are important, such as anointing the sick for Roman Catholics.

Native American

- First, determine what tribe(s) is involved.
- Attempt to determine the preferred term(s) to describe medical conditions and therapies?
- Anecdotes and metaphors are common means of communication - telling about a neighbor or relative may signify what the patient is experiencing.
- Do not interrupt a speaker; long pauses are part of communication
- A literacy assessment should be done - as well as determination of primary and secondary languages.
- Non-verbally, respect is usually communicated by lack of eye contact and keeping some distance in personal space.
- A light touch or handshake is usually appropriate. Soft tones and polite speech are appreciated. Humor, self-humor and willingness to tease reflect a positive atmosphere - but the patient or family should take the lead.
- Consents and decision-making should include asking patient if others will need to be consulted. Exactly who this may be will vary from tribe to tribe.
- Value is placed on personal autonomy. Illness may be viewed as a family matter and written consents may be viewed with distrust — based on personal and political history of misuse.
- Terminal illness discussions again vary among tribes. Some cultures may use information of prognosis to make preparations. Others prefer not to openly discuss such topics, as negative thoughts may hasten loss.
- Pain is generally under treated with Native Americans. Such general terms as "not feeling good" or "not right" may indicate discomfort. If they are not responded to with appropriate pain relief, the patient is unlikely to repeat request for assistance. Also complaints may be voiced to a family member who is then expected to relay this to the health care provider.
- Dyspnea, nausea, vomiting, constipation and diarrhea may be discussed in a matter-of-fact fashion.
- Efforts at self-care may be tried first using traditional Native medicine or in combination with Western medicine. Self-care and self-healing are important components to be in harmony with nature. Herbal treatment is common, including herbal teas.
- Other management of health may be done by ritual and mystical belief. Some Native American cultures have certain numbers which are sacred and other numbers which must be avoided.

Native American Continued

- If medicine bundles or pouches, prayer feathers and other amulets are present, do not casually move, examine or question about them.
- Some tribes avoid contact with the dying. Others will expect the immediate and extended family to be present, including small children. A positive attitude is usually maintained. Sadness and mourning will be expressed in a place away from the patient.
- Some tribal cultures will need an open window or will move the patient out of the home - perhaps to some facility. Others will orient the patient in a cardinal direction prior to death.
- When death has occurred, family may hug, touch, sing, stay close to the deceased. Wailing and shrieking may be outward signs of grieving.
- Care of the body will vary with culture and/or Christian beliefs. Tradition may dictate flexing the body, use of sweetgrass smoke or other purification rites. Some families will take the body in the home the night before burial to be cleansed and dressed to "spend the last night on the earth" and for visitation by family and friends. Time frames before the soul is believed to depart will vary, which may require delay in burial. Other cultures will avoid contact with the deceased and possessions.
- Denial and anger usually will be minimal. In some tribes outward signs of mourning and grief are considered natural and desirable for both sexes.
- There may be a year anniversary of the death in which feasting, remembrance and giving away of possessions may occur. In contrast with other tribes no overt mourning is culturally permissible. All possessions - even including the home - may be burned and no mention is directly made of the deceased.

Chinese

- Cantonese and Mandarin are the most common languages. Bilingualism in English varies with individuals. Elderly Chinese - particularly women - may be unable to read or write.
- Asking questions of health care workers may be seen as disrespectful; nodding is a sign of respect, politeness and may also signal understanding or agreement.
- Use formal address, particularly for elderly.
- The oldest male of family usually helps with medical decisions and consents. The caring role is usually the responsibility of a female in the household. The patient role is usually passive.

Chinese continued

- Be aware of nonverbal cues. Offer medications rather than waiting for patient to ask for them.
- Acupressure and acupuncture may be used - as may herbal remedies.
- Dyspnea, nausea / vomiting, constipation / diarrhea are viewed as yin/yang imbalance - and often treated with diet and herbal teas.
- Minor symptoms are often treated with food. Major symptoms and major illnesses may be ignored until advanced.
- Patients may be fatalistic and not want to discuss prognosis. Family may wish patient not be told - or prefer to tell the patient themselves.
- Special amulets, cloths, and ropes may be placed on the body. Incense may be used. Some families may choose to bathe the body after death.

Japanese

- Questions may be infrequent, deferring to the health care professional. Communication influenced by *enryo* (self-restraint in interactions with others) *gaman* (self-control and ability to endure) and *haji* (concept of shame/"face").
- Literacy in English varies. Nonverbal communication is typically quiet and polite. Facial expression controlled. Patients are respectful to elders and authority figures - with relatively little eye contact. Touching is uncommon. Nodding is common but not necessarily indicative of understanding or agreement. There is formal name use. Handshakes, smile or small bow may be appropriate.
- Family may "filter" information in the case of a serious or terminal illness. The family may be reluctant to share prognosis or diagnosis with the patient.
- Consult with family members (spouse, eldest son or daughter). Sick patients are cared for primarily by women.
- Patients may be stoic - offer pain management. Sick elders are traditionally cared for at home by eldest son's family.
- Cleanliness is important - along with preservation of modesty.

Cultural Sensitivity Guidelines

Somoan
- Most adults literate in Samoan and speak English to some degree.
- Non-verbally, politeness and deference are stressed. Touching is accepted as a sign of sincerity. Posture and relative height are important. Patients may be stoic - "god's will."
- First names preferred. A handshake is customary. Prognosis should be shared early.
- Massage is traditionally used for pain.
- Herbal medicines frequent. Traditional healer may be consulted.
- Ministers and family provide major support.
- The family usually will prepare body at death.
- Grief is displayed with feasting.

Black Americans
- Communication is primarily English with many traditional dialects, including black English - spoken mainly in inner cities.
- Silence may indicate lack of trust for the caregiver.
- Initially a handshake and formal address are appropriate.
- Consents and information sharing may be complicated by distrust engendered by personal and group history. It is best to have a family conference or talk with family elder or minister.
- The patient may have an oldest relative selectively reveal a poor prognosis.
- Expression of pain is usually open.
- Faith and root healers may be used in conjunction with biomedical resources; this information is frequently not shared with health care providers.
- Home remedies may be used first. Teas, herbs, warm compresses are common.
- Open and public emoting is expected, but this varies. Wailing common in immediate and/or extended family. Funerals are important event for grief - usually in religious context. Participation in funerals is expected by family with support by the community.
- The deceased is highly respected.

Depression Assessment Algorithm

Assessment Guidelines:
- Assess for vegetative signs and symptoms: insomnia, weight loss, appetite change, crying spells, suicidal ideation, lack of energy, inability to concentrate, anhedria, psychomotor retardation. Are signs and symptoms acute or chronic?
- Document stage of disease and functional status (See *Appendix*)
- Assess current medications
- Document stage of disease and functional status (See *Appendix*)
- Recent change in home setting/support system?
- Are there unmet spiritual needs or unfinished business? (See *Spiritual Assessment/Intervention Guide*)
- Is patient in pain? Any other unrelieved distressing symptoms? (See *Pain Algorithms*)
- Anxiety or agitation? (See *Anxiety or Agitation Treatment Algorithms*)
- Evidence of psychosis? (visual or auditory hallucinations)
- History of depression?
- Assess need for psychotherapy.
- History of seasonal affective disorder?
- Document *Quality of Life Scores* (See *Appendix*)
- Consider signs of dementia, especially in young patients.
- Perform mini-mental status examination (See *Appendix*)
- Document *FAST Score* (See *Appendix*)

Physician - Nurse - Pharmacist consultation for any etiology not addressed in algorithm

Implement appropriate non-pharmacologic interventions

Initiate *Depression Treatment Algorithm* and/or proceed to other associated algorithms

Non-Pharmacologic Interventions

• Encourage social work, chaplain, and volunteer visits if no other support systems in place • Initiate light therapy • Help facilitate a safe environment for the patient and caregiver, especially if the patient is contemplating self-harm • Counsel on sleep hygiene • Relaxation • Visualization • Hypnosis • Imagery • Therapeutic touch • Aromatherapy • Pet therapy • Educate patient and family regarding treatment options, medications and anticipated effects

Depression Treatment Algorithm

Signs and symptoms of depression

Sleep disturbance is not a major component of depression

Sleep disturbance is a significant component of depression and patient's ECOG $\geq$ 3

Initiate selective serotonin reuptake inhibitor*

- Paroxetine (Paxil) 20 mg PO QD (MDD 60 mg)
- Fluoxetine (Prozac) 20 mg PO QD (MDD 80 mg)
- Sertraline (Zoloft) 50 mg PO QD (MDD 200 mg)
- Venlafaxine (Effexor) 25 mg PO TID (MDD 375 mg)
- Nefazodone (Serzone) 100 mg PO BID (MDD 600 mg)
- Citalopram (Celexa) 20 mg PO QD (MDD 60 mg)

*For frail or elderly, consider initiating at 1/2 the dose and titrate to effect. Reassess at two and six weeks

- Amitriptyline* (Elavil) 50 mg PO Q HS. Titrate up every 3 - 5 days by 50 mg to 150 mg. Reassess at 4 - 6 weeks for efficacy. Advise patient of side effects, especially orthostatic hypotension; consult physician prior to initiating if any cardiac disease present.
- Trazodone* (Desyrel) 50 mg PO Q HS. Titrate up every 3 - 5 days by 50 mg as needed. Average dosage range is 150 mg to 400 mg. (MDD 400 mg)

*For frail or elderly, consider initiating at 1/2 the dose and titrate to effect. Reassess at two and six weeks

Physician - Nurse - Pharmacist consultation. Consider initiating a psychostimulant (See *Adjuvant Medication Guide in Appendix*). Initiate mental health consultation (psychiatrist, psychologist, psychiatric nurse or mental health worker) as indicated

Diarrhea Assessment

Assessment Guidelines
- See *Bowel Assessment and Treatment Algorithm*
- Assess for fecal impaction
- Assess for food intolerance (milk, spices, rich)
- Current or recent medications? (side effect of medications?, recent antibiotics?, antacid use?)
- Disease process? (i.e. colitis, history of hemoccult positive stool)
- Recent history of radiation treatments or chemotherapy?
- Assess for overuse/abuse of laxatives
- Past history of chronic diarrhea
- Assess for pain and cramping
- Assess for infectious etiology (i.e. food or water contaminants). Document stool hemoccult; consider stool culture and sensitivity.
- History of abdominal surgery? Consider bowel obstruction. (See *Adjuvant Medication Guide-Visceral Pain* in the *Appendix*)
- Assess for presence of skin breakdown (See *Candidiasis Perineal Algorithm* and *Skin Care Algorithm*)

Initiate *Diarrhea Treatment Algorithm* and/or proceed to other associated algorithms

Physician-Nurse-Pharmacist consultation for etiology not addressed in this algorithm

Implement appropriate non-pharmacologic interventions

Non-Pharmacologic Interventions

- Educate patient and family on treatment options, medications and anticipated effects • Educate patient and family that some acute diarrheal episodes are self-limited and do not require specific therapy • Consider modification of the diet (clear liquids for a day, avoid dairy products) • Attend to perineal skin care (apply powder or dry padding to prevent irritation) • Avoid stimulants such as caffeine and nicotine.

Diarrhea Treatment Algorithm

Clear liquids for 24 hours, advance to low residue diet

Relief

No Relief

Advance diet as tolerated; avoid spices, fats, rich foods, and stimulants such as caffeine or nicotine

Initial options
- Kaopectate 60 - 120 mL PO after each loose stool for 48 hours or loperamide (Imodium AD) 1 tab PRN loose stools (not to exceed 8 tabs/24 hours)
- Calcium polycarbophil (Mitrolan) 1 gram PO QID
- Metamucil - 5 - 15 cc mixed with water PO BID. For patients receiving tube feeding, adding 7 grams per liter has been shown to eliminate diarrhea.

No Relief

Discontinue loperamide (Imodium AD). Add diphenoxylate HCl with atropine (Lomotil) 1 tab after each loose bowel movement. MDD 8 tabs. Adjust dose to patient's response.*

No Relief

Physician–Nurse–Pharmacist consultation for further orders. For secretory diarrhea, consider low dose octreotide 50 - 100 µg Q 8 hrs SQ.

Relief

Advance diet as tolerated

* - For AIDS patients, consider metronidazole (Flagyl) 500 mg PO BID
  - If malabsorption is contributing to diarrhea, pancrease 2 caps prior to meals

Dyspnea Assessment

Assessment Guidelines

- Assess stage of disease process. Other associated symptoms? [i.e. ascites, (See *Ascites Algorithm*), pleural effusion, lung metastases, hepatomegaly, pneumothorax]
- Document respiratory rate, pulse and blood pressure
- Infectious etiology?
- Anxiety component (See *Anxiety Treatment Algorithm*)
- Assess fluid status (congestive heart failure, renal disease, hepatic disease)
- Hemoglobin level - document baseline hemoglobin level
- Oximetry - when appropriate
- If the patient is a smoker, educate patient regarding the risk of oxygen use while smoking
- History of pulmonary disease?
- History of cardiac disease?
- Unmet spiritual needs? (*Consult chaplain,* See *Spiritual Assessment Guide*)
- Document a *Quality of Life Score* (See *Appendix*)
- Document a functional and/or *FAST Score* (See *Appendix*)

Initiate *Dyspnea Algorithm* and/or proceed to other associated algorithms

Physician-Nurse-Pharmacist consultation for etiology not addressed in this algorithm

Implement appropriate non-pharmacologic interventions

Dyspnea Assessment
Non-Pharmacologic Interventions

• Educate patient and family regarding treatment options,
medications and anticipated effects • Educate patient and
family on positioning techniques to facilitate chest expansion
• Elevate head of bed (pillows, bed support) • Cool room
environment • Wet cloth on face • Use fan in room to
improve circulation of air • Rearrange home environment to
minimize patient exertion • Breathing exercises • Hypnosis
• Visualization • Relaxation techniques • Emotional support
and reassurance • Eliminate allergens and smoke • Fluid
restriction diet • Low Sodium Diet if indicated

Nebulized Opioids

Use of Nebulized Opioids

- Nebulized opioids should not be used for pain relief because
  of low systemic bio-availability (5%). The putative receptors
  are on larger airways so the particle size is immaterial.

- Most patients prefer a mouthpiece rather than a mask

- Start with morphine sulfate 4 mg diluted in 3 mL saline OR
  hydromorphone 2 mg in 3 mL saline. If not effective, then
  double the concentration.

- Nebulize with air or oxygen up to 8 L/min for 10 minutes or
  until most of the solution has disappeared

- Repeat Q 4 h ATC and Q 1 h PRN

Dyspnea Treatment Algorithm

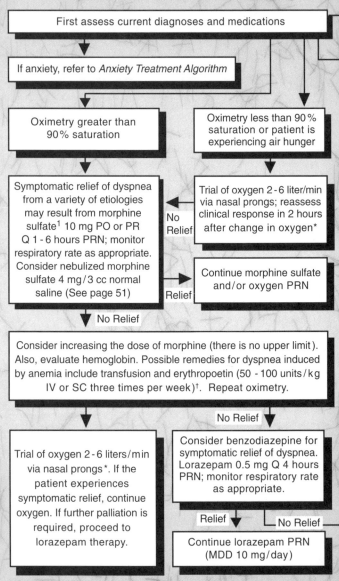

First assess current diagnoses and medications

If anxiety, refer to *Anxiety Treatment Algorithm*

Oximetry greater than 90% saturation

Oximetry less than 90% saturation or patient is experiencing air hunger

Symptomatic relief of dyspnea from a variety of etiologies may result from morphine sulfate[1] 10 mg PO or PR Q 1 - 6 hours PRN; monitor respiratory rate as appropriate. Consider nebulized morphine sulfate 4 mg / 3 cc normal saline (See page 51)

Trial of oxygen 2 - 6 liter/min via nasal prongs; reassess clinical response in 2 hours after change in oxygen*

No Relief

Continue morphine sulfate and / or oxygen PRN

Relief

No Relief

Consider increasing the dose of morphine (there is no upper limit). Also, evaluate hemoglobin. Possible remedies for dyspnea induced by anemia include transfusion and erythropoetin (50 - 100 units / kg IV or SC three times per week)[†]. Repeat oximetry.

No Relief

Trial of oxygen 2 - 6 liters/min via nasal prongs*. If the patient experiences symptomatic relief, continue oxygen. If further palliation is required, proceed to lorazepam therapy.

Consider benzodiazepine for symptomatic relief of dyspnea. Lorazepam 0.5 mg Q 4 hours PRN; monitor respiratory rate as appropriate.

Relief

No Relief

Continue lorazepam PRN (MDD 10 mg/day)

*Consider humidified oxygen for prolonged use. †See *Fatigue Algorithm*

www.Intelli-card.com

If dyspnea is due to congestive heart failure (crackles/rales, peripheral edema), initiate therapy with diuretics, nitrates and oxygen. Monitor urine output, daily weights and presence of peripheral edema.

If bronchospasm (audible wheezing) assess current medications and oxygen therapy

Start beclomethasone (Vanceril) inhaler 1-2 inhalations 3-4 times/day and/or albuterol 1-2 inhalations Q 4-6 hours PRN (consider spacer). Switch to nebulizer treatment if needed

No Relief

Add ipratropium bromide (Atrovent) 1-2 inhalations 3-4 times per day

No Relief

Physician–Nurse–Pharmacist consultation. Consider oral steroids or antibiotics. Consider nebulized morphine sulfate 4 mg/3 cc normal saline (See page 51 for nebulized MS; also refer to *Adjuvant Medication Guide* in *Appendix* and *Cough Algorithm*)

- Furosemide (Lasix) 20-40 mg PO for one dose. If effective, continue furosemide 20-40 mg PO daily or BID
- Initiate supplemental potassium therapy (start with potassium chloride 20 mEq PO daily).
- If there is no diuresis with furosemide 80 mg PO BID, then Physician-Nurse-Pharmacist consultation
- Nitrates: Nitropatch 0.2-0.4 mg/hr topically daily
- Oxygen[2]: If the patient's 0_2 saturation is below 90%, consider supplemental oxygen 2-6 liters/min by nasal canula. Alternatively, use a ventimask (5 liters per min)
- Is the patient a candidate for home BiPAP?

If there is relief, continue

No Relief

Physician-Nurse-Pharmacist consultation for further orders.

[1] Morphine sulfate may be palliative in patients with dyspnea even if there is no pain. If there is any question about suppression of the respiratory drive, then a physician-nurse consultation is indicated. Careful dosing with naloxone (Narcan) may be appropriate.

[2] Heliox may also be therapeutic in selected patients.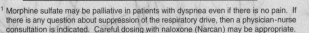

Falls Assessment

Assessment Guidelines:
- Document vital signs including postural vital signs
- Assess mental status (See *Mini-Mental Status Exam in Appendix*)
- Assess ability to actively move all extremities
- Assess for presence of deformity; check distal pulses for asymmetry; assess for decreased sensation, pallor, skin temperature
- Assess for presence of pain (See *Pain Algorithms*)
- Assess for possible etiology of falls (patient slipped, weakness, loss of consciousness, seizure, drug related, cardiac arrhythmia)
- Document stage of disease and functional status (See *Appendix*)
- Assess frequency of toileting needs
- Document *Quality of Life Scale* (See *Appendix*)
- Document *FAST Score* (See *Appendix*)

Initiate *Falls Treatment Algorithm* and/or proceed to other associated algorithms

Physician-Nurse-Pharmacist consultation for etiology not addressed in this algorithm

Determine probable etiology and eliminate further risk. Implement appropriate non-pharmacologic interventions

Non-Pharmacologic Interventions

• Discuss with patient and family treatment options, medications, and anticipated effects • Use side rail while in bed • Use cane or walker (patient should demonstrate reasonable proficiency) • Catheter • Ambulation with assistance • Time outings when patient most alert and energetic • Take extra time to move from recumbant to upright posture • Mobility alarms • Bedpan • Helmet • Bedside commode

Falls Treatment Algorithm

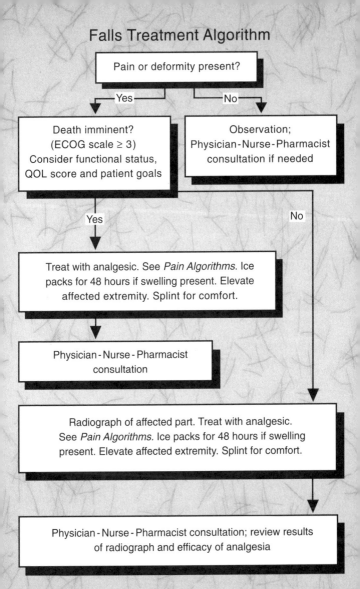

Pain or deformity present?

Yes → Death imminent? (ECOG scale ≥ 3) Consider functional status, QOL score and patient goals

No → Observation; Physician-Nurse-Pharmacist consultation if needed

Yes → Treat with analgesic. See *Pain Algorithms*. Ice packs for 48 hours if swelling present. Elevate affected extremity. Splint for comfort.

→ Physician-Nurse-Pharmacist consultation

No → Radiograph of affected part. Treat with analgesic. See *Pain Algorithms*. Ice packs for 48 hours if swelling present. Elevate affected extremity. Splint for comfort.

→ Physician-Nurse-Pharmacist consultation; review results of radiograph and efficacy of analgesia

Fatigue Assessment

- Document stage of disease and functional status? (See *PPS, ECOG/Karnofsky, FAST Score* in *Appendix*)
- What is the duration and intensity of fatigue over the last six months (use a 0-10 scale and time line)
- Document Quality of Life score (See *FACT Score, Linear Analog Score, or MVQOL score* in *Appendix*)
- Patient's description of fatigue: tired, loss of energy, exhausted
- Explore impact of fatigue on personal well being, family dynamics, work, intimacy, social life and future orientation.
- What activities or circumstance seem to counteract the fatigue?
- Are patient's pain and other distressing physical symptoms controlled?
- Is patient anemic? Is so, what type of anemia is present (See *Fatigue Treatment Algorithm*)
- Has the patient benefited from prior transfusions?
- Does the patient have an anemia of chronic disease?
- Has the patient undergone recent or ongoing myelosuppressive chemotherapy?
- Does the patient have underlying liver disease and/or coagulopathy?
- Is there evidence of blood loss?
- Is hemolysis present: autoimmune, traumatic, drug induced?
- Is tumor infiltration of bone marrow present?
- Are nutritional deficiencies in erythropoietin cofactors, such as iron, B-12, folate present? If so, document prior levels and therapies.
- Review medications for potential drug-induced anemia? (e.g. zidovidine)
- Assess other nutritional status; consider a nutritional consult. Is there evidence of underlying gastrointestinal malabsorption?
- For patients with anemia or nutritional deficiencies, document hemoglobin, platelets, reticulocyte count, albumin, and protein.
- What is patient's appetite? (See *Appetite Loss Algorithm*)
- Is infection or fever present? (See *Fever Assessment Algorithm* and associated algorithms)
- Is patient depressed or anxious? (See *Depression Algorithm* or *Anxiety Assessment and Treatment Algorithm*) Document the MMSE (mini-mental status examination - see *Appendix*)
- Is sleep disturbance a major factor? Document normal sleep/wake/rest patterns (See *Sleep Disturbance Assessment and Treatment Algorithm*)
- Is patient able to exercise? Would patient benefit from physical therapy or occupational therapy?

Fatigue Assessment continued on next page ▶

Fatigue Assessment

Continued from previous page

- What is patient's HIV status?
- What other underlying medical conditions exist? Have hypothyroidism, adrenal insufficiency or hormonal deficiencies been considered?
- Would patient benefit from oxygen therapy? (See *Dyspnea Algorithm*)
- Are there underlying psychological stressors or spiritual issues not yet addressed? (See *Psychosocial and Spiritual Assessment Guides*)
- Are environmental factors an issue?

Initiate *Fatigue Treatment Algorithm* and/or proceed to other associated algorithms

---

Physician - Nurse - Pharmacist consultation for etiology not addressed in this algorithm

Implement appropriate non-pharmacologic interventions

Non-Pharmacologic Interventions

- Educate patient and caregivers regarding adverse effects of prolonged bedrest and excessive inactivity • Attempt exercise if feasible • Establish realistic goals for daily living • Help patient establish activities and priorities within individual limitations • Provide guidance on the balance between rest and activity • Encourage keeping a journal to identify fatigue patterns • Schedule important activities during most energetic periods of the day • Hospital bed • Mechanical support as needed • Physical therapy and occupational therapy as tolerated by the patient • Eliminate nonessential activities
- Support self care interventions regularly • Pet therapy
- Psychotherapy, support groups, spiritual counselors, if indicated

Fatigue Treatment Algorithm

Determine the etiology of the fatigue. Is there anemia?

For anemic patients classify type of anemia; document impact on function and QOL (Quality of Life); use QOL linear analog scale or MVQOL Score for interval assessments

Hypoproliferative anemias (deficient storage or utilization of iron)

- **Iron deficiency**:
- Document source of blood loss, hemolysis vs inadequate intake or absorption
- Document recent ferritin level < 20 ng/ml or < 50 ng/ml plus transferrin saturation of < 0.08
- Peripheral blood smear: microcytic, hypochromic red blood cells

Treatment: Identify source of blood loss (check stool hemoccults) and control if possible. For suspected GI source, verify that GI prophylaxis is in place (See *Gastrointestinal Prophylaxis Treatment Algorithm*); skin or mucosal ulcerations (See *Skin Care Treatment Guidelines* and *Mucositis Treatment Algorithm*); consult physician as needed
Begin trial of ferrous sulfate 325 mg daily; constipation prevention measures are recommended.

- **Anemia of chronic disease** (inability of reticulocyte endothelial system to reuse iron from red blood cell breakdown)
- Document associated illness; e.g. cancer, renal failure, chronic infection, etc.
- Has thalassemia been ruled out?
- Document recent ferritin levels > 50 ng/ml, and low serum iron and transferrin levels
- Peripheral blood smear: microcytic or normocytic, hypochromic red blood cells (no sideroblasts or basophilic stippling)

Treatment: Trial of ferrous sulfate 325 mg PO QD, consider trial of erythropoietin (Epoetin alpha) 100 units/kg three times per week for one month; if no increase in Hb (hemoglobin) >1 g/dl after one month, discontinue therapy; if an increase in hemoglobin is documented, increase dose to 150 units/kg TIW with Hb check monthly until Hb >12. Reassess every other week patient goals, stage of disease and quality of life using linear analog scale (See *Quality of Life Scores in Appendix*)

- **Stem cell dysfunction**: aplastic anemia or myelodysplastic syndrome
- Document invasion of bone marrow by tumor or other etiology per hematologist-oncologist; was a bone marrow biopsy done?
- Peripheral blood smear: pancytopenia for aplastic anemia or nucleated red cells, megakaryocytes, metamyelocytes for myelodysplastic syndrome

Treatment: Consider Quality of Life scores, prior efficacy of transfusions. If appropriate, transfuse or try erythropoetin therapy as done in anemia of chronic disease above.

Fatigue Treatment Algorithm

For other causes of fatigue, go to the next page

Ineffective erythropoiesis anemias
- **B12 deficiency** (pernicious anemia)
- Document serum vitamin B12 levels < 100 pg/ml or urine methylmalonic acid and homocysteine elevated
- What symptom complex is suggestive of pernicious anemia?
- Peripheral blood smear: macrocytic red blood cells, pancytopenia, hypersegmented PMN's

Treatment: Vitamin B12 100 mg IM monthly until stores repleted

- **Folate deficiency**
- Document serum folate level < 2 ng/ml
- Is patient an alcoholic or on medications that impair absorption/metabolism?
- Is there a neoplastic, inflammatory, or hemolytic process?
- Always assess B12 status prior to initiating therapy.

Treatment: Folate 1 mg PO QD or 1 prenatal vitamin QD

- **Sideroblastic anemia (acquired) or DiGuglielmo's syndrome**
- Document bone marrow or peripheral blood smear with sideroblasts
- Is there underlying neoplastic, inflammatory, or drug ingestion contributing?
- Always assess B12 and folate status as well

Treatment: Consider a trial of pyridoxine 200 mg tid if not tried previously. If no rise in Hb > 1 g/ml in 1 month, discontinue.

- **Thalassemia** - document history

Hemolytic anemias

Autoimmune and microangiopathic
- For elderly, recent documentation of positive Coomb's test or cold agglutinins
- Usually associated with a lymphoproliferative disorder, collagen vascular disease or drug ingestion; microangiopathic hemolysis may lead to disseminated intravascular coagulation, especially in the terminal process
- Peripheral blood smear: microspherocytes

Treatment: supportive therapy; avoid cold temperatures; based on functional status (ECOG > 3) and Quality of Life score, may benefit from iron, folate or B12 replacement

(patient often with prior splenectomy, cyclophosphamide and steroid trial prior to coming on to a palliative care service)

Fatigue Treatment Algorithm

Investigate other causes of fatigue
(continued from the previous page)
Consider some of the following possibilities:

For patients with Sleep Deprivation,
see *Sleep Disturbance Algorithm*.

Patient with endocrine disorder
- Physician-Nurse-Pharmacist consultation to determine therapy
  for an endocrine disorder such as adrenal insufficiency,
  hypothyroidism, or hormonal imbalance

Patient with infection
- See related algorithms that suggest empiric antibiotics (*Bladder Spasm Algorithm, Cough Algorithm, Dyspnea Algorithm, Fever Algorithm*)
- If choice of therapy is not clear with other algorithms, Physician-Nurse-Pharmacist consultation

Fatigue Treatment Algorithm

Fatigue related to medications (iatrogenic)
- Attempt to taper or discontinue medications that may be contributing to a sense of fatigue
- If opioid induced sedation is contributing, see *Opioid Induced Sedation Algorithm*.

For patients with a mood disorder, see *Depression Algorithm*, *Anxiety Algorithm*, and *Agitation Algorithm*; see *Adjuvant Medication Guide in Appendix*.

If non-pharmacologic interventions and other pharmacologic interventions fail to improve the patient's sense of fatigue, reassess patient and caregiver expectations.
Physician - Nurse - Pharmacist consultation

For patients with respiratory compromise, consider the following interventions:
- Optimize oxygenation (If indicated, see *Dyspnea Algorithm*)
- Treat any underlying pulmonary infection (See *Cough Algorithm* for antibiotic suggestions)

Fever Assessment

Assessment Guidelines

- Assess potential sources of infection -- wound infection, viral syndrome, UTI (*See Bladder Algorithm*), pharyngitis or mucositis (See *Candida Algorithm* and *Mucositis Algorithm*), GI or GU symptoms, pulmonary symptoms (See *Dyspnea/Cough Algorithm*), skin breakdown (See *Skin Care Algorithm*)
- Address pain relief measures if indicated (See *Pain Guidelines*)
- CNS dysfunction? Document MMSE (Mini-Mental Status Examination - See *Appendix*)
- Decreased fluid intake? Discuss the patient's directive on use of intravenous hydration.
- Document stage of disease and functional status (See *Appendix*)
- Document *Quality of Life Score* (See *Appendix*)
- Document *FAST Score* (See *Appendix*)

Initiate *Fever Algorithm* and/or proceed to other associated algorithms

Physician–Nurse–Pharmacist consultation for etiology not addressed in this algorithm

Implement appropriate non-pharmacologic interventions

Non-Pharmacologic Interventions

- Cooling measures (disrobe, tepid water bath, fan in room, ambient temperature control, push clear liquids) • Mouth care as needed • Discuss with patient and family the treatment options, medications and anticipated effects

Fever Treatment Algorithm

Document presence of fever.
Is an infection present?

 Yes

No

Source of infection is suspected by history or exam.
- For bladder symptoms, see *Bladder Algorithms*.
- For respiratory symptoms, see *Cough Algorithm* and *Dyspnea Algorithm*.
- For skin breakdown, see *Skin Care Guidelines and Treatment Algorithm*.

Physician-Nurse-Pharmacist consultation for possible antibiotic therapy and diagnostic work up

Treat symptomatically for end stage disease (ECOG rating ≥ 3-4). Physician-Nurse-Pharmacist consultation

Increase fluids as tolerated. Treat symptomatically as directed by the patient's advanced directive. Suggestions: fan, cool wash cloths, moisten mouth and lips

- Acetaminophen (Tylenol) 650 mg PO/PR Q 3-4 hours PRN temperature over 100° orally.
- Ibuprofen (Motrin) 400-600 mg PO Q 6 h PRN
- Indomethacin (Indocin) 50 mg suppository PR Q 8 h PRN
- See Non Opioid Analgesic and NSAID table in Appendix)

Relief

No Relief in 48 hours

Treat as needed

Physician-Nurse-Pharmacist consultation

Gastroesophageal Reflux Assessment

Assessment Guidelines
- History of peptic ulcer disease or other bowel disease?
- Is there post prandial acid brash in pharynx?
- Is there post prandial belching?
- Is there post prandial chest pain (usually a retrosternal burning or pain)?
- Is there pain when swallowing? Worse with liquids or solids?
- Does the patient or family report relief with antacids?
- Current use of non-steroidal antiinflammatory agents or steroids?
- Is nausea present? (*See Nausea Treatment Algorithm*)
- History of gastric upset with administration of medications?
- History of neuromuscular disease?
- History of diabetes with known diabetic gastroparesis?
- Document mental status (MMSE in *Appendix*)
- History of gall bladder or pancreas problems?
- History of food intolerance?
- History of Helicobacter pylori? (See *Appendix* for treatment)
- History of abdominal surgery?
- History of recent drug or alcohol misuse?
- Review dietary habits (caffeine, chocolates, nicotine)
- Change in stool color, consistency, or caliber?
- Assess for psychosocial or spiritual stressors (*See Psychosocial and Spiritual Assessment Guidelines*)
- Document stage of disease, QOL score, and functional status (See *Appendix*)

Initiate *Gastroesophageal Reflux Algorithm* and/or proceed to other associated algorithms

Physician-Nurse-Pharmacist consultation for etiology not addressed in this algorithm

Implement appropriate non-pharmacologic interventions

Non-Pharmacologic Interventions

- Educate patient and family on treatment options, medications, and anticipated effects • After meals, remain sitting (avoid reclining for at least one hour) • Elevate head of bed • Bland diet • Small frequent meals • Avoid offending foods (especially caffeine, nicotine, alcohol) • Consider staying NPO until treatment is initiated • Modify environment to reduce stress.

Gastroesophageal Reflux Treatment Algorithm

For any acute mid-epigastric discomfort, consider
- Maalox plus (15-30 mL) PO PRN; may mix with 5 mL viscous lidocaine 2% or 5 mL benzocaine 20% PO PRN
- Sucralfate (Carafate) 1 gm PO AC & HS up to QID

Misoprostol (Cytotec)* 100-200 µg PO TID with food and QHS (MDD 800 µg) plus proton pump inhibitor

Proton pump inhibitor:
- Omeprazole (Prilosec) 20 - 40 mg PO Q day (capsules)
- Lansoprazole (Prevacid) 15 - 30 mg PO Q day before eating (capsules)

Consider H_2 blocker
- Ranitidine (Zantac) 150 - 300 mg PO QHS (tablet or liquid)
- Cimetidine (Tagamet) 200 - 800 mg QHS (tablet or liquid)
- Famotidine (Pepcid) 20 - 40 mg PO HS (tablet or liquid)
- Nizatidine (Axid) 150 - 300 mg PO HS (pulvules)

Metoclopramide (Reglan) 10 mg PO Q 6 - 8 hours after meals and at bedtime may also be effective

 Relief   Relief   No Relief

Continue as needed. Reassess at regular intervals. Attempt to taper therapy as clinical findings improve.

Physician - Nurse - Pharmacist consultation. Would the patient benefit from a gastroenterology consultation or empiric therapy for Helicobacter Pylori? (See *Appendix*)

---

* Consider modifying the bowel program to anticipate diarrhea as a side effect of misoprostol

For elderly, discontinue NSAIDs; switch to opioid for pain control. See *Non Opioid Analgesic Chart* in *Appendix*.

When patients on nonsteroidal antiinflammatory agents, consider switching to cyclooxygenase II inhibitor (eg. celecoxib [Celebrex])

Gastrointestinal Assessment

Assessment Guidelines
- History of peptic ulcer disease or other bowel disease?
- Are there symptoms of gastroesophageal reflux or pain with swallowing? (See *Gastroesophageal Reflux Algorithm* or *Oral Candidiasis Algorithm*)
- Current use of nonsteroidal antiinflammatory agents or steroids?*
- Is nausea present? (*See Nausea Treatment Algorithm*)
- History of gastric upset with administration of medications?
- Review dietary habits (caffeine, chocolate, nicotine)
- History of gall bladder or pancreas problems?
- History of food intolerance?
- History of Helicobacter pylori? (Treatment guide in *Appendix*)
- History of abdominal surgery?
- History of neuromuscular disease?
- History of diabetes with diabetic gastroparesis?
- History of recent drug or alcohol abuse?
- Change in stool color, consistency, or caliber?
- Assess for psychosocial or spiritual stressors (*See Psychosocial and Spiritual Assessment Guidelines* in *Appendix*)
- Document the patient's mental status (MMSE in *Appendix*)
- Assess patient's age and weight for proper medication dosing

*(Relative contraindications to NSAIDS in elderly)

Initiate *GI Prophylaxis Algorithm* and/or proceed to other associated algorithms

Physician-Nurse-Pharmacist consultation for etiology not addressed in this algorithm

Implement appropriate non-pharmacologic interventions

Non-Pharmacologic Interventions

- Educate patient and family on treatment options, medications, and anticipated effects •Bland diet •Small frequent meals
- Avoid offending foods (especially caffeine, nicotine, alcohol)
- Consider staying NPO until treatment is initiated •Modify environment to reduce stress.

Gastrointestinal Treatment Algorithm

Misoprostol (Cytotec)* 100 - 200 µg PO TID with food and QHS (MDD 800 µg) plus proton pump inhibitor

Proton pump inhibitor:
- Omeprazole (Prilosec) 20 - 40 mg PO Q day (capsules)
- Lansoprazole (Prevacid) 15 - 30 mg PO Q day before eating (capsules)

Consider H2 blocker:
- Ranitidine (Zantac) 150 - 300 mg PO QHS (tablet or liquid)
- Cimetidine (Tagamet) 200 - 800 mg QHS (tablet or liquid)
- Famotidine (Pepcid) 20 - 40 mg PO HS (tablet or liquid)
- Nizatidine (Axid) 150 - 300 mg PO HS (pulvules)

Metoclopramide (Reglan) 10 mg PO Q 6 - 8 hours after meals and at bedtime may also be effective.

No Relief

- Sucralfate (Carafate) 1 gm PO AC & HS up to QID - or -
- Antacid over-the-counter 30 mL PO Q 4-6 hrs

No Relief

For any acute epigastric discomfort, consider Maalox plus (15 - 30 mL) mixed with viscous lidocaine 2% 5 mL or benzocaine 20% 5 mL PO PRN

Relief

Relief

No Relief

Continue as needed. Reassess at regular intervals. Attempt to taper therapy as clinical findings improve.

Physician-Nurse-Pharmacist consultation. Would the patient benefit from a gastroenterology consultation or empiric therapy for Helicobacter Pylori? (See *Appendix*)

Note:
- For elderly, discontinue NSAIDs; switch to opioid for pain control. See *Non Opioid Analgesic Guide* in *Appendix*.
- For patients on nonsteroidal antiinflammatory agents, consider switching to cyclooxygenase II inhibitor (eg. celecoxib [Celebrex]).

* Consider modifying the bowel program to anticipate diarrhea as a side effect of misoprostol

Headache Assessment

- What was the patient's age at the onset of headaches?
- Is this a sudden onset headache? (Consider vascular event such as subarachnoid hemorrhage or intracranial hemorrhage)
- Assess frequency and duration of the headache
- What is the site of the headache?
- What is the time of onset of the headache?
- Are there associated signs or symptoms (nausea, photophobia, visual complaints, sleep disorder, motor or sensory changes)?
- Are there aggravating and relieving factors?
- Is there concomitant substance misuse (alcohol, nicotine, cocaine)?
- Has there been a history of trauma?
- Is there a history of migraine headache or other recurrent headache syndrome?
- Are there additional medical illnesses (malignancy [consider cerebral metastases], immunocompromised, hypertension)?
- Assess current medications (blood thinners, chronic use of analgesics).
- CNS dysfunction? Document MMSE (Mini-Mental Status Examination - See *Appendix*)
- Document stage of disease and functional status (See *Appendix*)
- Document *Quality of Life Score* (See *Appendix*)
- Document *FAST Score* (See *Appendix*)
- History of depression? (See *Depression Algorithm*)
- Assess psychosocial stressors and spiritual needs (See *Psychosocial and Spiritual Assessment Guides*)
- Assess for allergic conditions. Are there signs and symptoms of sinus trouble?
- Assess oxygenation. Record pulse oximetry. Are there indications for supplemental oxygen? (See *Dyspnea Algorithm*)
- Assess for presence of meningitis (fever, headache, stiff neck, altered mental status) or sinusitis
- See examination points on the next page

Initiate *Headache Algorithm* and/or proceed to other associated algorithms

Physician-Nurse-Pharmacist consultation for etiology not addressed in this algorithm

Implement appropriate non-pharmacologic interventions

Headache Assessment

Examination Points

Vital signs - temperature, pulse, blood pressure, respiratory rate

Constitutional assessment - Does the patient look ill or in distress? Is the patient mentally alert or is there decreased mental status?

Head/Scalp - Inspect the scalp and face for a skin eruption (shingles). In elderly patients, palpate the temporal arteries and note any tenderness.

Ears - Evaluate the external auditory canals and tympanic membranes for signs of infection.

Eyes - Is the intraocular pressure normal? Are pupils equal and reactive? Is nystagmus present? Is there redness? Assess extraocular movement, anterior chamber and fundoscopic exam.

Cranial nerve function - Evaluate cranial nerves

Face - Assess for tenderness in scalp, temples, occiput, sinuses, and tympanomandibular joints

Mouth and pharynx - Assess dentition and tympanomandibular joint.

Neck - Assess for suppleness, masses, and areas of tenderness

Neurologic examination - Assess and document if the patient is alert and oriented, cranial nerves 2 - 12 intact, motor examination shows 5/5 strength, sensory examination is intact, and pathologic reflexes are absent. Document mini mental status examination (See *Appendix*)

Non-Pharmacologic Interventions

• Avoidance of loud noise, strong smells, flashing lights, missed or delayed meals, stress, possible offending foods such as nicotine, caffeine, cheese, chocolate, citrus fruits and alcohol
• Quiet environment • Positioning of patient for comfort
• Elevate head of bed when increased intracranial pressure is known or suspected • Hot and cold compresses • Would patient benefit from OT/PT? • Teach visualization, self-hypnosis
• Music therapy • Massage • Humor • Relaxation techniques
• Water therapy • Biofeedback • TENS unit • Meditation
• Acupressure • Acupuncture • Aromatherapy • Therapeutic touch • Abstain from substance abuse • Exercise if possible
• Pet therapy • Educate patient and family regarding treatment options, medications and anticipated effects

Headache Treatment

See *Pain Algorithms*
Titrate based upon clinical condition and response

↓

For specific headache syndromes such as migraine headaches, see *Specific Headache Treatment Regimens* in *Appendix*

↓

For patients with sleep disturbance, see *Sleep Disturbance Algorithm*

↓

If there is associated nausea, see *Nausea Algorithm*

↓

If there is known or suspected increased intracranial pressure consider dexamethasone 2 - 10 mg PO, IM, PR QID for three days. Taper dexamethasone as determined by the clinical response. (See Adjuvant Medication Guide in Appendix)

↓

With documented hypoxemia, administer supplemental oxygen as needed to improve pulse oximetry to 90% or higher (See *Dyspnea Algorithm*)

↓

Physician - Nurse - Pharmacist consultation for discussion of etiologies and therapies not addressed in this algorithm (meningitis, sinusitis, dental pain, intracerebral metastases, drug rebound, drug withdrawal, hypertension, glaucoma, intracranial hemorrhage).

Consider initiating prophylactic medications to prevent headaches (See *Headache Prophylactic Medications* in the *Appendix*).

Consider specific treatments for headache syndromes (See *Specific Headache Medications and Regimens* in *Appendix*)

Notes

Hiccough Assessment

Assessment Guidelines
- Assess for presence of gastrointestinal disease
  (See *Gastroesophageal Reflux Algorithm* and *Gastrointestinal Treatment Algorithm*)
- Consider irritation of the diaphragm due to gastric distension, hepatomegaly, irritation of the phrenic nerve, or progession of disease
- Consider metabolic abnormalities (especially with renal failure)
- Assess for neurologic and psychologic illnesses
- Document stage of disease, QOL and functional status
  (See *Appendix*)

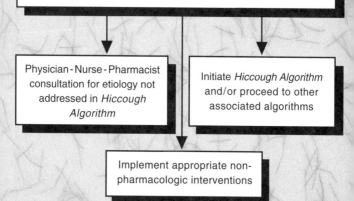

Physician - Nurse - Pharmacist consultation for etiology not addressed in *Hiccough Algorithm*

Initiate *Hiccough Algorithm* and/or proceed to other associated algorithms

Implement appropriate non-pharmacologic interventions

Non-Pharmacologic Interventions

• Educate patient and family regarding treatment options, medications and anticipated effects • Bag rebreathing • Have patient drink liquids slowly • Offer patient a teaspoon of sugar to hold in the mouth and then swallow • Nasopharyngeal stimulation with cotton swab or NG tube • Keep patient as comfortable as possible • NG tube if gastric distension present • Keep patient NPO for 24 hrs • Distraction • Cool compresses to eyes

Hiccough Treatment Algorithm

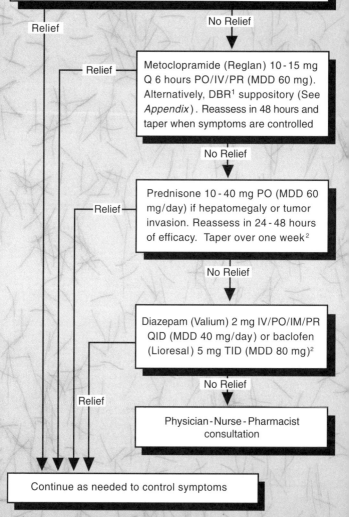

Chlorpromazine (Thorazine) 25 - 50 mg Q 6 hours PO,IV, or PR. (MDD 200 mg)   Reassess at 48 hours. Monitor BP carefully, especially if used IV.

Relief

No Relief

Relief

Metoclopramide (Reglan) 10 - 15 mg Q 6 hours PO/IV/PR (MDD 60 mg). Alternatively, DBR[1] suppository (See *Appendix*). Reassess in 48 hours and taper when symptoms are controlled

No Relief

Relief

Prednisone 10 - 40 mg PO (MDD 60 mg/day) if hepatomegaly or tumor invasion. Reassess in 24 - 48 hours of efficacy. Taper over one week[2]

No Relief

Diazepam (Valium) 2 mg IV/PO/IM/PR QID (MDD 40 mg/day) or baclofen (Lioresal) 5 mg TID (MDD 80 mg)[2]

No Relief

Relief

Physician - Nurse - Pharmacist consultation

Continue as needed to control symptoms

[1]DBR = Decadron (4 mg) - Benadryl (25 mg) - Reglan (10 mg)
[2]See *Adjuvant Medication Guide* in the *Appendix*

Mucositis Assessment

Assessment Guidelines
- Assess oral cavity including tongue, gingiva, mucous membranes, lips and saliva
- Assess voice quality and swallowing ability
- Assess oral hygiene practices (Is patient rinsing mouth frequently with plain water? Is patient brushing?)
- Assess nutrition and fluid intake
- Assess recent chemotherapy or radiation treatments
- Assess medications (i.e. sulfa therapy that could lead to drug induced mucositis)
- Assess dentition and fit of dentures
- Is patient at risk for graft versus host disease? (i.e. previous bone marrow transplant)
- Assess pain – (See *Pain Algorithm*)
- Is there oral candidiasis? (See *Oral Candidiasis Algorithm*)
- Is there evidence of bacterial overgrowth (cellulitis, papillitis)?
- Assess for psychosocial and spiritual stressors (See *Psychosocial* and *Spiritual Assessment Guidelines*)

Physician-Nurse-Pharmacist consultation for etiology not addressed in *Mucositis Algorithm*

Initiate *Mucositis Treatment Algorithm* and/or proceed to other associated algorithms

Implement appropriate non-pharmacologic interventions

Non-Pharmacologic Interventions

•Educate patient and family on treatment options, medications and anticipated effects •Artificial saliva •Lip balm •Brush teeth frequently using soft brush (≥3 times per day) •Encourage hydration •Rinse mouth frequently with non-irritating, non-alcoholic mouth wash (glyoxide peroxide or cetyl pyridium in glycerin) •Avoid nicotine and alcohol intake •Recommend soft mechanical diet and cool, non-irritating foods •Educate patient and family regarding symptoms requiring more aggressive treatment

Mucositis Treatment Algorithm

- Isotonic saline or sodium bicarbonate rinses Q 1-2 hours while awake for 48 hours (1.5 teaspoons salt in 1 quart of water -or- 1.25 teaspoons of sodium bicarbonate in 1 pint of water).
- For mucosal debris, consider trial of 1:4 ratio of water/peroxide rinses followed by saline rinse.
  (See *Pain-Step One Treatment Algorithm* for pain relief)
- For oral candidiasis, see *Oral Candidiasis Algorithm*
- Discontinue medications known to cause mucositis (i.e. sulfa drugs)

- Peridex rinses QID
- Sucralfate (Carafate) slurry swish and spit as needed. Patient may hold in mouth 3-5 minutes or allow to dribble down throat if there are signs or symptoms of esophageal involvement
- Lidocaine/diphenhydramine/antacid (1:1:1) or benzocaine gel or solution 20% (Hurricane) 5 mL swish and swallow AC and Q 6-8 H for 3 days. Hold in mouth 3-5 mins. (Caution in patients with impaired gag reflex – swish and spit). Consider use of other topical anesthetics

For discrete ulcers use:
- Amlexanox oral paste 5% (Aphthasol) - apply QID for ten days. Apply when aphthous ulcers begin, to achieve better results
- Zilactin gel topically to ulcerations
- Viscous lidocaine 2% applied with cotton tip applicator to discrete oral ulcerations may also provide transient relief
- Benzocaine 20% oral gel (Hurricane) - apply topically PRN

If signs of gingival papillitis, cellulitis or other signs of bacterial infection, initiate 7-10 day course of antibiotics
- Amoxicillin/clavulanate (Augmentin) 875 mg PO BID
- Clindamycin (Cleocin) 300-600 mg PO QID
- Metronidazole (Flagyl) 500 mg PO TID

Relief	No Relief
Continue as needed. Reassess at 7 days and PRN.	Physician-Nurse-Pharmacist consultation for further orders

Nasal Congestion Assessment

Assessment Guidelines

- History of other associated symptoms? (allergy, upper respiratory infection, cough [See *Cough Algorithm*])
- Allergy assessment - Animals in house; Dust mites; Is air filtered?
- Onset? Duration?
- Is air humidified?
- History of recurrent symptoms?
- Consider overuse of over-the-counter nasal sprays with rebound phenomenon (e.g. Afrin, neosynephrine)
- Current medications?
- Pain in sinuses and/or purulent secretions from nasal passages?
- Is epistaxis present?

Physician-Nurse-Pharmacist consultation for etiology not addressed in *Nasal Congestion Treatment Algorithm*

Initiate *Nasal Congestion Treatment Algorithm* and/or proceed to other associated algorithms

Implement appropriate non-pharmacologic interventions

Non-Pharmacologic Interventions

- Warm packs to face • Warm, humidified air • Encourage fluid intake, especially hot beverages Ointment to nasal mucosa • Gentle, infrequent nose blowing • Eat hot, spicy foods • Hot showers • Elevate head of bed • Mouth care • Exercise may improve rhinitis • Eliminate household allergens with air filters • Frequent cleaning • Remove pets from living area if acceptable to patient • Educate patient and family regarding etiology and treatment options, medications, and anticipated effects

Nasal Congestion Treatment Algorithm

- Normal saline nasal drops/spray (Ocean) frequently/PRN
- Ponaris - half dropper each nostril PRN or with cotton tip applicator
- Antibiotic ointment to dry mucosa TID

Relief → Continue as needed

No Relief → No history of hypertension

If patient has hypertension

Discontinue after 3 days of total therapy

Pseudoephedrine (Sudafed) 15 - 30 mg tabs 1 - 2 PO Q 4 - 6 hours PRN

Relief

Treatment options:
- Oxymetazolone (Afrin) Nasal Spray 0.05% 2 - 3 sprays BID
- Phenylephrine (Neosynephrine) Nasal Spray 0.25%, 0.50% or 1.0% 1 - 2 sprays each nostril Q 4 - 6 hours

Monitor blood pressure

No Relief

No Relief

Relief

Beclomethasone Nasal spray 1 - 2 sprays Q 12 hours

Continue for 5 - 7 days. Reassess.

No Relief

Relief

Physician–Nurse–Pharmacist consultation for further orders. Consider methylprednisolone (Depo-Medrol) 40 - 80 mg IM or antibiotic for suspected infection.*

Continue ≤3 weeks. Reassess.

*See Cough Algorithm for antibiotic guidelines

Nausea & Vomiting Assessment

Assessment Guidelines   Consult *Adjuvant Medication Guide* in *Appendix*
- Assess pattern of nausea/vomiting
- Assess for presence of unrelieved pain (See *Pain Algorithm*)
- Assess for constipation and/or GI stasis
  (See *Bowel Program Algorithm*)
- Assess for presence of anxiety and other triggering
  factors (See *Anxiety Algorithm*)
- Assess oral cavity for evidence of thrush
  (See *Oral Candidiasis* or *Mucositis Algorithm*)
- Assess for medication side effects/toxicity
- Assess for symptoms of increased intracranial pressure*
- Assess for symptoms of motion sickness
- Do you suspect bowel obstruction or pseudo obstruction?*
- Hypercalcemia? (breast cancer/bone metastases)
- Electrolyte disturbances?
- Assess diet for offending foods
- Does anyone else in family display flu symptoms?
- Recent history of chemotherapy?
- Suspect gastritis (burning, mid epigastric pain)?
  (See *Gastroesophageal Reflux Algorithm* and
  Gastrointestinal Treatment Algorithm)

Physician-Nurse-Pharmacist consultation for etiology not addressed in algorithm

Implement appropriate non-pharmacologic interventions

Initiate *Nausea/Vomiting Algorithm* and/or proceed to other associated algorithms

*See Adjuvant Medication Guide

Nausea & Vomiting Non-Pharmacologic Interventions

- Educate patient and family on treatment options, medications and anticipated effects • Set realistic goals and discuss treatment options with patient/family and consequences of treatment versus no treatment • Distraction • Good oral hygiene
- Eliminate offending foods, tastes or smells • Acupressure
- Explore patients belief system regarding etiology of nausea
- Diet changes - Low fat, small frequent feedings, non-gas forming foods • Visualization/relaxation techniques • Liquid diet for next 24 hours to rest the GI tract and allow the anti-emetics a chance to work • Experiment with sour foods such as lemons, sour pickles, hard sour candy, or lemon sherbert
- Experiment with a variety of eating patterns • Avoid eating or drinking for 1-2 hours after vomiting • Eat cold foods or those served at room temperature such as a sandwich, cottage cheese, cereal, desserts to avoid odors of fat foods • Utilize a clear liquid diet to reduce nausea - apple juice, cranberry juice, broth, ginger ale, popsicles, gelatin, tea or cola drinks • Sip liquids slowly. • Sip off a spoon; this prevents gulping • Bland foods - mashed potatoes, apple sauce, sherbert, crackers, toast • Ginger - capsules, tablets, candy, tea

Nausea and Vomiting Treatment Algorithm

Gastritis - See
Gastrointestinal Treatment

← If possible, establish cause

↓

Nausea associated with increased intracranial pressure

↓

Physician-Nurse-Pharmacist consultation for steroid order. Consider trial of dexamethasone (Decadron) 2 mg PO TID. Titrate dexamethasone based upon clinical results. Reassess every 24 - 48 hours.
Consult Adjuvant Medication Guide in Appendix

↓

Nausea associated with motion or excessive pulmonary secretions

↓

Transderm scopolamine (Transderm Scop) [3] topically for 72 hours; or scopolamine hydrobromide (Scopine) 0.4 mg tablets; or atropine sulfate [4] 0.4 mg

↓

If no decrease in pulmonary secretions add iodinated glycerol 20 drops in water QID or potassium iodide (PIMA) 5 - 10 mL PO TID [5]

↓

Physician - Nurse - Pharmacist consultation if no relief after one week

[1] DBR = Decadron (4 mg) - Benadryl (25 mg) - Reglan (10 mg)
[2] RDA = Reglan (50 mg) - Decadron (10 mg) - Ativan (2 mg)
    See *Appendix* for Suppository Preparation instructions
[3] Alternatives to scopolamine patches include scopolamine time released capsules, hyoscyamine preparations (Cystospaz - M, Levsinex Timecaps, Levsin drops), promethazine transdermal gel (0.25 - 0.5 mL) of a 50 mg/mL gel per compounding pharmacist.
[4] Atropine is contraindicated in patients with glaucoma or asthma.
[5] Avoid PIMA in patients with hyperthyroidism or renal disease

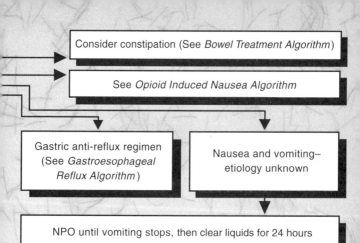

Consider constipation (See *Bowel Treatment Algorithm*)

See *Opioid Induced Nausea Algorithm*

Gastric anti-reflux regimen (See *Gastroesophageal Reflux Algorithm*)

Nausea and vomiting– etiology unknown

NPO until vomiting stops, then clear liquids for 24 hours

- Prochlorperazine (Compazine) 10 mg PO Q 6 hours, 25 mg rectal suppository Q 12 hours PRN, transdermal gel 0.25 - 0.5 mL of 50 mg/mL gel
- Odansetron (Zofran) 8 mg (tablet or oral solution) PO BID. Intravenous odansetron is given 32 mg over 15 minutes.
- Granisetron (Kytril) 10 µg/kg intravenous over 5 minutes. Alternatively 1 mg PO Q 12 hours

Consult *Adjuvant Medication Guide* in *Appendix*

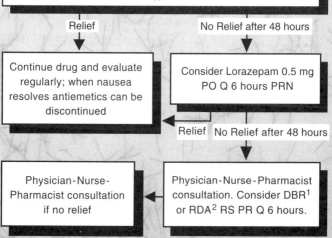

Relief

No Relief after 48 hours

Continue drug and evaluate regularly; when nausea resolves antiemetics can be discontinued

Consider Lorazepam 0.5 mg PO Q 6 hours PRN

Relief   No Relief after 48 hours

Physician-Nurse-Pharmacist consultation if no relief

Physician-Nurse-Pharmacist consultation. Consider DBR[1] or RDA[2] RS PR Q 6 hours.

Opioid Induced Nausea Treatment Algorithm

- Has initial opioid therapy just started?
  – or –
- Has opioid dose just been increased?
  – or –
- Is the patient on appropriate bowel regimen?

 No

Look for causes other than the opioid such as physiologic changes or other medications.
See *Nausea Assessment* guidelines.

Consult Adjuvant Medication Guide in Appendix

Yes

If symptoms suggest opioid induced labyrinthian dysfunction (motion sickness symptoms) medications include:

- Prochlorperazine (Compazine) 25 mg PR Q 12 hrs PRN
- Prochlorperazine (Compazine) 10 mg PO or IM Q 6 hours PRN
- Meclizine (Antivert) 25 - 50 mg PO Q 8 hrs PRN
- Transderm scopolamine (Transderm Scop) one patch Q 72 hours. Alternatives to scopolamine patches include scopolamine time released capsules, hyoscyamine preparations (Cystospaz-M, Levsinex Timecaps, Levsin drops), promethazine transdermal gel (0.25 - 0.5 mL) of a 50 mg/mL gel (pharmacist with authorization to compound can create gel)

Reassess in 48 - 72 hours. Tolerance should develop in 3 - 7 days at a stable opioid dose.
Attempt to taper as nausea subsides

If symptoms suggest opioid induced reduced gastric motility, try metaclopramide (Reglan) 10 mg PO/PR/IV QID AC -or- cisapride (Propulsid) 10 mg PO TID

For assessment and non-pharmacologic interventions, see *Nausea and Vomiting Assessment*

Notes

Opioid–Induced Sedation Assessment

Assessment Guidelines:
- Has opioid therapy recently been started or increased?
- Are adjuvants and other pain modalities optimized?
- Assess patient's sleep pattern in the past few weeks (See *Sleep Disturbance Algorithm*)
- Is effective pain relief contributing to sedation and relaxation? Do other sedative–hypnotics need to be tapered?
- Review patient's medications for other contributing causes and possible drug interactions
- Assess for depression (See *Depression Algorithm*)
- Assess respiratory status (See *Dyspnea* or *Cough Algorithm*)
- Is concomitant pulmonary disease present?
- Consider disease progression; CNS involvement?
- Is hepatic/renal disease or GI malabsorption interfering with drug metabolism or elimination?

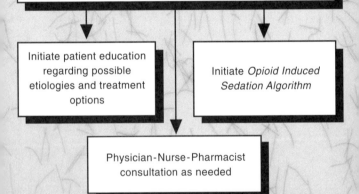

Initiate patient education regarding possible etiologies and treatment options

Initiate *Opioid Induced Sedation Algorithm*

Physician-Nurse-Pharmacist consultation as needed

Non-Pharmacologic Interventions

- Oral intake of stimulants such as caffeinated beverages
- Sleep hygiene counselling • Increase stimulating activities
- Patient and family education regarding treatment options, medications and anticipated side effects

Opioid–Induced Sedation Treatment Algorithm

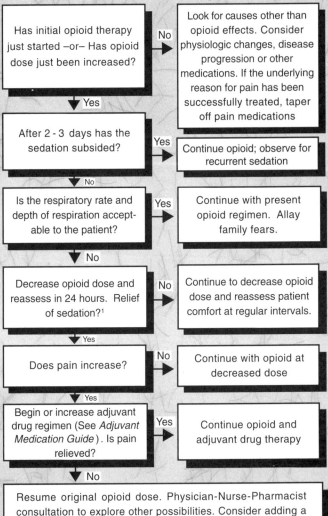

Has initial opioid therapy just started –or– Has opioid dose just been increased? → **No** → Look for causes other than opioid effects. Consider physiologic changes, disease progression or other medications. If the underlying reason for pain has been successfully treated, taper off pain medications

↓ **Yes**

After 2 - 3 days has the sedation subsided? → **Yes** → Continue opioid; observe for recurrent sedation

↓ **No**

Is the respiratory rate and depth of respiration acceptable to the patient? → **Yes** → Continue with present opioid regimen. Allay family fears.

↓ **No**

Decrease opioid dose and reassess in 24 hours. Relief of sedation?[1] → **No** → Continue to decrease opioid dose and reassess patient comfort at regular intervals.

↓ **Yes**

Does pain increase? → **No** → Continue with opioid at decreased dose

↓ **Yes**

Begin or increase adjuvant drug regimen (See *Adjuvant Medication Guide*). Is pain relieved? → **Yes** → Continue opioid and adjuvant drug therapy

↓ **No**

Resume original opioid dose. Physician-Nurse-Pharmacist consultation to explore other possibilities. Consider adding a stimulant (i.e. caffeine, methylphenidate, pemoline, dextroamphetamine)[2]

[1]See *Pearls for Analgesic Titration*
[2]See *Adjuvant Medication Guide* regarding opioid induced narcolepsy

Pain Assessment Algorithm – Step One

- Location of pain (See *Pain Assessment form* in *Appendix*)
- Quality of pain (dull, sharp, aching, shooting)
- Intensity of pain (pain rating using 0-10 scale)
- Aggravating factors (things that bring on or make pain worse)
- Alleviating factors (things that diminish pain or make it better)
- Associated symptoms? - nausea, anorexia, sleep disturbance (See *Associated Algorithms*)
- Liver or renal dysfunction? (*Physician-Nurse-Pharmacist consultation*)
- Past history of gastritis or recent GI bleeding?
- Assess for psychosocial and spiritual stressors (See *Psychosocial and Spiritual Assessment Guidelines*)
- Are cultural barriers present? (See *Cultural Sensitivity Guidelines*)
- Document a *QOL Score* (See *Appendix*)
- Document stage of disease and functional status (See *Appendix*)

Implement appropriate non-pharmacologic interventions

Initiate *Step One* of *Pain Treatment Algorithm* and/or proceed to other associated algorithms

Physician-Nurse-Pharmacist consultation for:
• Etiology not addressed in algorithm • Patient allergic to recommended medications • Patient has history of gastritis or recent gastrointestinal bleeding (See *GI or GERD Algorithms*)

Non-Pharmacologic Interventions

• Positioning of patient for comfort (hospital bed in home, eggcrate mattress, alternating pressure mattress) • Support affected painful area • Hot and cold applications • Would patient benefit from OT/PT or dietician consultation? • Consider other home assistance devices • Teach visualization, self-hypnosis • Music therapy • Massage • Humor • Meditation • Relaxation techniques • Water therapy • Biofeedback • Aromatherapy • TENS unit • Acupressure • Acupuncture • Therapeutic touch • Pet therapy • Educate patient and family on treatment options, medications and anticipated effects

Pain Treatment Algorithm - Step One
(Mild to moderate pain - Pain scale 1 - 3)

If possible, establish probable cause of pain

↓

Consider the need for weak opioid while pain is initially being brought under control (treatment options):
- Acetaminophen 500 mg Q 4 hours PO or PR ATC (MDD 4000 mg)
- Celecoxib (Celebrex)* 100 mg PO BID (MDD 400 mg)
- Choline Magnesium Trisalicylate PO ATC (usually 1500 mg loading dose then 500 mg PO BID - TID; MDD 4000 mg; tab or liquid)
- Ibuprofen 200 mg 2 - 3 tabs Q 4 hours PO ATC (MDD 4200 mg)
- Indomethacin 25 mg 2 - 3 times/day PO or PR ATC (MDD 200 mg)

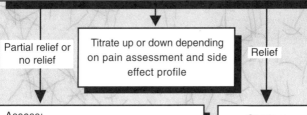

Partial relief or no relief | Titrate up or down depending on pain assessment and side effect profile | Relief

Assess:
- Appropriate dosing schedule
- Patient adherence with ATC dosing
- Need for upward titration
- Need for change to different non opioid analgesic (See *Appendix*)
- Assess need for adjuvant medications (See *Adjuvant Medication Guide* in *Appendix*)
- Consider initiating *GI treatment protocol* for projected chronic NSAID use.

Continue medications and reassess at regular intervals

No Relief

Relief

Continue medications and reassess at regular intervals

Advance to *Pain Algorithm Step Two*

---

* Cyclooxygenase II inhibitors (celecoxib) with diminished gastrointestinal side effects, may be preferred to cyclooxygenase I inhibitors.

Pain Assessment Algorithm - Step Two

- Location of pain (See *Pain Assessment Form* in *Appendix*)
- Quality of pain (dull, sharp, aching, shooting)
- Intensity of pain (pain rating using 0-10 scale)
- Aggravating factors (things that bring on or make pain worse)
- Alleviating factors (things that diminish pain or make it better)
- Associated symptoms? - nausea, anorexia, sleep disturbance (See *associated algorithms*) Is there a need to increase bowel regimen?
- Liver or renal dysfunction? (*Physician-Nurse consultation*)
- Past history of gastritis or recent GI bleeding?
- Has progression of disease been addressed? Would patient benefit from initiation of steroids?
- Are spiritual and psychosocial needs being addressed? (See *Spiritual and Psychosocial Assessment Guidelines*)
- Are there physician attitude barriers or knowledge/skill issues to address?
- Document *QOL Score* (See *Appendix*)
- Are cultural barriers present? (See *Cultural Sensitivity Guidelines*)
- Document stage of disease and functional status (See *Appendix*)

| Notify physician that the therapy is advancing to *Step Two* of the *Pain Management Algorithm* | Implement appropriate non-pharmacologic interventions |

Physician-Nurse-Pharmacist consultation if pain rating is consistently ≥ 5 on a scale of 0-10 for greater than 24 hours in spite of repeated upward titrations. Consider advancing to *Step Three* (See *Pearls for Analgesic Titration* in *Appendix*)

Non-Pharmacologic Interventions

- Positioning of patient for comfort (hospital bed in home, eggcrate mattress, alternating pressure mattress) • Support affected painful area • Hot and cold applications • Would patient benefit from OT/PT or dietician consultation? • Consider other home assistance devices • Teach visualization, self-hypnosis • Music therapy • Pet therapy • Massage • Humor • Meditation • Relaxation techniques • Water therapy • TENS unit • Biofeedback • Acupressure • Acupuncture • Aromatherapy • Therapeutic touch • Educate patient and family regarding treatment options, medications and anticipated effects

Pain Treatment Algorithm-Step Two

(Moderate to Severe Pain - Pain Scale 4 - 6)

- Hydrocodone 5 mg/APAP 500 mg: 1 - 2 tabs Q 4 hours (*MDD 8 tabs*)
- Oxycodone 5 mg (*tab or liquid*) PO Q 6 hours ATC
- Oxycodone CR (Oxycontin) 10 - 20 mg RS Q 12 hours ATC
- Fentanyl patch 25 µg/hour Q 72 hours (*MDD limited by skin surface area and effectiveness*)
- Will need breakthrough medication with fentanyl patch. Suggested breakthrough medications: oxycodone 5 - 10 mg Q 4 - 6 hours; oxycodone (20 mg/mL) 10 mg PO Q 12 hours; fentanyl oralet (10 - 15 µg/kg/dose) 200 - 1600 µg/day

Titrate analgesic up or down based on pain assessment and continue non-opioid started in *Step One*. Continue adjuvants or add adjuvants as needed. Consult *Adjuvant Medication Guide in Appendix*.

 Relief   Partial Relief or No Relief

Continue medications. Reassess at regular intervals. Titrate as necessary to maintain pain control and minimize side effects

Assess:
- Appropriate dosing schedule
- Patient adherence with ATC dosing
- Need for upward titration
- Need for change to different opioid
- Assess need for adjuvant medications
  (See *Adjuvant Medication Guide* in *Appendix*)
- Does patient need GI prophylaxis?
- Is bowel protocol in place?
  (See *GI, GERD, Bowel Algorithm* if indicated)

 No Relief

Continue medications and reassess at regular intervals

Proceed to *Pain Algorithm Step Three*; notify the physician that the treatment is advancing to next level

Pain Assessment Algorithm - Step Three

- Location of pain (See *Pain Assessment Form* in *Appendix*)
- Quality of pain (dull, sharp, aching, shooting)
- Intensity of pain (pain rating using 0 -10 scale)
- Aggravating factors (bring on or make pain worse)
- Alleviating factors (diminish pain or make it better)
- Associated symptoms? - nausea, anorexia, sleep disturbance (See *associated algorithms*) Is there a need to increase bowel regimen?
- Liver or renal dysfunction? (*Physician - Nurse consultation*)
- Past history of gastritis or recent GI bleeding?
- Has progression of disease been addressed? Would patient benefit from initiation of steroids or other adjuvants?
- Has a medication review been performed to avoid polypharmacy?
- Assess patient directive on the use of more aggressive routes of opioid delivery
- Are there physician attitude barriers or knowledge/skill issues to address?
- Are spiritual and psychosocial needs being addressed? (See *Spiritual and Psychosocial Assessment Guidelines*)
- Are cultural barriers present? (See *Cultural Sensitivity Guidelines*)
- Document QOL Score and functional status (See *Appendix*)

Implement appropriate non - pharmacologic interventions

- Initiate *Step Three* of *Pain Algorithm*
- Physician - Nurse - Pharmacist consultation if pain rating is consistently ≥5 on a scale of 0 - 10 for greater than 24 hours in spite of repeated upward titrations.

Non - Pharmacologic Interventions

- Positioning of patient for comfort (hospital bed in home, eggcrate mattress, alternating pressure mattress) • Support affected painful area • Hot and cold applications • Would patient benefit from OT/PT or dietician consultation? • Consider other home assistance devices • Music therapy • Teach visualization, self-hypnosis • Massage • Pet therapy • Humor • Meditation • Relaxation techniques • Water therapy • Biofeedback • TENS unit • Acupressure • Acupuncture • Aromatherapy • Therapeutic touch • Educate patient and family regarding treatment options, medications and anticipated effects.

[1] The authors recommend that the initial dose of oral hydromorphone be given in doses lower than the equianalgesic chart would indicate.

[2] See PCA Assessment and Pain Management Options table. Is the patient a candidate for epidural analgesics/clonidine, neurolytics, palliative radiation therapy, or chemo-therapy? Consider midazolam, pentobarbital, or thiopental drip if end stage (See *Terminal Agitation Algorithm*); review patient directive for care

Pain Treatment Algorithm - Step Three
(Severe Pain Treatment Algorithm - Pain Scale 7 - 10)

Establish probable cause

↓

Starting dose should be at least equianalgesic to previous analgesic agent. Titrate analgesic up or down based on pain assessment and continue non-opioid and adjuvants as started in step two. (See *Equianalgesic Chart*) Consult *Pain Management Options* and *Adjuvant Medication Guide* in *Appendix*)

↓

Suggested opioid naive patient dosages:
- Morphine 10 mg Q 2-4 hours PO, SL, PR (*tablet, liquid, suppository*); 2-4 mg Q 1 hour for SC or IV ATC (*no ceiling dose*)
- Hydromorphone (Dilaudid)[1] 1-3 mg Q 3-4 hours PO, 3 mg PR; 1-2 mg SC or IV ATC (*no ceiling dose*)
- These are recommended starting doses; doses need to be individualized according to pain assessment
- Titrate up or down based on pain assessment (See *Equianalgesic Chart* and *Pearls for Analgesic Titration* in the *Appendix*)

Patients requiring opioids for persistent pain often require a longer acting opioid. Consider transdermal fentanyl (Duragesic) 25 µg/hour Q 72 hours -or- controlled release morphine - (MS Contin) 15-30 mg BID PO, PR ATC (*no ceiling dose*)

↓ Partial Relief or No Relief   ↓ Relief

Assess: • Appropriate dosing schedule • Patient adherence with ATC dosing • Need for upward titration • Need for change to different opioid • Need for adjuvant medications • Need for GI prophylaxis? • Is bowel protocol in place?	Continue medications and document reassessments at regular interval. Titrate as necessary to maintain pain control
	Do in depth pain assessment. Physician−Nurse−Pharmacist consultation for alternative pain relief measures [2]

Relief   No Relief →

Continue medications and document reassessments at regular intervals

PCA Pain Assessment Algorithm
PCA = Patient Controlled Analgesia

Criteria for instituting PCA
- Patient no longer able to swallow
- Patient is unable to tolerate side effects of oral medications*
- Rectal route not convenient, appropriate, or acceptable to caregiver
- Patient has erratic GI absorption of medications
- Pain not well controlled with oral medications even after multiple upward titrations and maximal use of adjuvants
- Transdermal pain medications with breakthrough medications (oral or transmucosal) are not effective
- Are there family barriers or cultural barriers to traditional care? (See *Cultural Sensitivity Guidelines*)
- Are there physician attitude barriers, knowledge or skill issues to address?

Route of Administration
- Subcutaneous route is preferred in the home setting except if patient already has a vascular access device (such as a groshong, PICC, or Port)
- Consider EMLA cream (lidocaine 2.5% + prilocaine 2.5%) be applied for 30 minutes prior to establishing an IV

- Starting dose of morphine or hydromorphone (Dilaudid) should be equianalgesic to current oral dose of opioid (See conversion formula and equianalgesic chart). Meperidine (Demerol) is inappropriate for chronic pain management.
- Physician–Nurse–Pharmacist consultation if patient with documented allergy to morphine and hydromorphone (Dilaudid).
- Consider methadone, levorphanol, or transdermal fentanyl with oral transmucosal fentanyl citrate (See opioid conversion table in the *Appendix*)

- Usual concentration of morphine and hydromorphone (Dilaudid) is 10 mg/mL. More concentrated solutions are used when the hourly rate exceeds 10 mg/hr. Concentration is calculated according to the hourly rate.
- SC infusion should not exceed 2 mL/hr.
- PCA bolus (rescue or breakthrough dose) = 25% - 50% of the hourly rate every 10 - 15 minutes.

*See *Pain Management Options* in *Appendix*

PCA Titration of Opioids

PCA = Patient Controlled Analgesia

TITRATION PARAMETERS:
- Calculate the past 24 hour opioid requirement
  (hourly rate x 24 **plus** total 24 hour boluses in mg given in 24 hours)
- Divide 24 hour opioid requirement by 24. This equals the new hourly rate
- New rescue bolus dose = 25% - 50% of the new hourly rate
  NOTE: Titration should occur at any time patient's pain is out of control (i.e. pain rating is $\geq 3/10$ on scale of 0-10 or the patient is using ≥ 3 oral breakthrough doses in 24 hours)

No Relief   Relief

- For pain rating consistently $\geq 3/10$ on scale of 0-10 for greater than 24 hours, continue titrations until pain score ≤ 3 or using $\leq$ three breakthrough dosages in 24 hours
- See *Pearls for Analgesic Titration* in *Appendix*

Continue to assess and titrate up or down PRN to maintain optimal pain control

Physician–Nurse–Pharmacist consultation. Consider switching to another opioid. Consider cross tolerance. Would the patient benefit from neurolytics, palliative radiation therapy, chemotherapy, epidural or intrathecal infusion?
(See *Pain Management Options* in the *Appendix*)

PROCEDURE FOR CHOOSING AN EQUIANALGESIC DOSE OF A NEW OPIOID

- **Use the equianalgesic dose chart (Appendix)**
- **Formula for conversions:**
  1. Add up the total 24 hour dose requirement of each current opioid which is being given.

     If both parenteral and oral doses were used, calculate a separate total for each.
  2. Divide each 24 hour dose requirement by the equianalgesic dose listed in the equianalgesic dose chart for the current opioid and current route of administration. The number obtained is called the *equianalgesic unit*.
  3. Multiply the *equianalgesic unit* by the equianalgesic dose of the new opioid (considering the new route).

Example: **Change route of administration from IV to PO:**

A patient is on fentanyl IV infusion of 0.02 mg (20 µg/hr) and will convert to an oral morphine regimen.

  1. The total 24 hr requirement of IV fentanyl is calculated as follows: 0.02 mg x 24 hours = 0.48 mg (480 µg)
  2. First convert IV fentanyl to IV morphine. The equianalgesic dose on the chart is 0.1 mg. Divide 0.48 mg by 0.1 = 4.8 (equianalgesic units).
  3. Now convert IV morphine to PO form. 4.8 x 30 (equianalgesic dose) = 144 mg/24 hours. For BID dosing (144/2 = 72 mg), order 75 mg (60 + 15 mg tabs) of MS Contin; alternatively, order (144/6 = 24 mg) 25 mg Q 4 hours.

Example: **Change route of administration from IV to PO:**

A patient has been receiving IV morphine 1 mg/ hour with 0.5 mg boluses Q 10 min. The patient has used 10 boluses in the past 24 hours. Convert to oral morphine; giving controlled release morphine orally twice a day.

  1. **The total 24 requirement of morphine:**
     Morphine dose in 24 hours = 24 mg + 5 mg = 29 mg.
  2. **Convert to equianalgesic units:**
     The equianalgesic dose on the chart is 10 mg, therefore 29 divided by 10 = 2.9 (*equianalgesic units*)
  3. **Convert to oral dose of morphine:**
     2.9 x 30 (equianalgesic dose of PO morphine) = 87 mg per 24 hours. Divide this by 6 and the morphine dose is equal to 14.5 mg Q 4 hour ATC. Alternatively, divide 87 mg/24 hours by 2 and the controlled release morphine dose = 43.5 mg Q 12 h. Controlled release morphine (MS Contin) can be given as 45 mg (30 mg tab plus 15 mg tabs) BID.

Example:
Change to different opioid:

A patient is on oxycodone/acetaminophen (Percocet) 2 tabs Q 4 hours ATC and has not been well controlled over the last 3 - 4 days. The patient will start on oral controlled release morphine.

1. **The total 24 requirement of oxycodone plus acetaminophen:**
   The total 24 hour requirement has been oxycodone 60 mg plus acetaminophen 3900 mg.

2. **Convert to equianalgesic units:**
   The equianalgesic dose for oxycodone on the chart is 30 mg, therefore 60 divided by 30 = 2 equianalgesic units.

3. **Convert to oral dose of morphine:**
   2 x 30 (equianalgesic dose of PO morphine) = 60 mg. Divide by 2 doses = 30 mg controlled release morphine Q 12 h.

4. **Continue acetaminophen:**
   The acetaminophen would be continued at the present dose or switched to an NSAID. (See *Pain Algorithm-Step One* , Also see *Adjuvant Medication Guide* and *Non Opioid Analgesic Table* in the *Appendix*)

5. **Breakthrough medication:**
   Also, provide a dose for breakthrough or incident pain. This could be 10 mg immediate release morphine Q 2 - 4 hours PRN. (Recommended breakthrough dose is 25 - 33% of Q 12 hour controlled release oral dose)

- In the above examples other multidimensional factors need to be assessed.
- Reassess for efficacy of dose and presence of side effects at regular intervals.

Pruritus Assessment

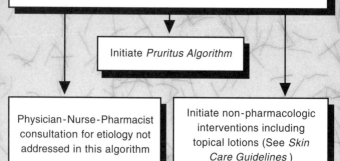

Assessment Guidelines:
- Onset, frequency, duration, and intensity
- Aggravating factors?
- Alleviating factors?
- Presence of scratch marks? Rash?
- Presence of other skin conditions?
- Presence of signs and symptoms of infection?
- Presence of liver or renal failure?
- Identify actual or potential causes of pruritus
- Review medications to rule out drug eruption

Initiate *Pruritus Algorithm*

Physician-Nurse-Pharmacist consultation for etiology not addressed in this algorithm

Initiate non-pharmacologic interventions including topical lotions (See *Skin Care Guidelines*)

Non-Pharmacologic Interventions

- Cool compresses • Hypoallergenic aqueous soaps (oatmeal) or aqueous moisturizers (Dove, Aveeno) • Trim fingernails
- Relaxation techniques • Sodium bicarbonate baths • Positive imagery • Lubricants if skin is dry • Cotton gloves at night to minimize excoriations • Loose fitting clothing and bedcovers
- Cotton clothing soaked in cornstarch and water • Pat skin (no rubbing or scratching)

Pruritus Treatment

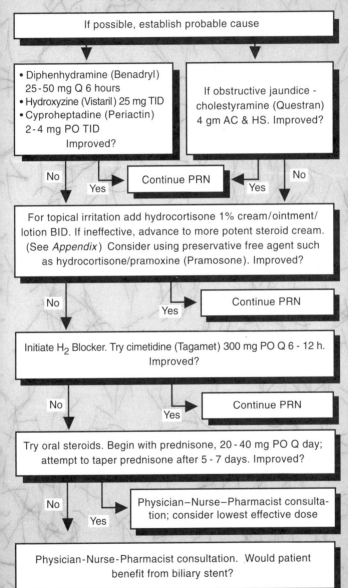

If possible, establish probable cause

- Diphenhydramine (Benadryl) 25 - 50 mg Q 6 hours
- Hydroxyzine (Vistaril) 25 mg TID
- Cyproheptadine (Periactin) 2 - 4 mg PO TID

Improved?

If obstructive jaundice - cholestyramine (Questran) 4 gm AC & HS. Improved?

No → Continue PRN ← No
Yes → Continue PRN ← Yes

For topical irritation add hydrocortisone 1% cream/ointment/lotion BID. If ineffective, advance to more potent steroid cream. (See *Appendix*) Consider using preservative free agent such as hydrocortisone/pramoxine (Pramosone). Improved?

No
Yes → Continue PRN

Initiate H₂ Blocker. Try cimetidine (Tagamet) 300 mg PO Q 6 - 12 h. Improved?

No
Yes → Continue PRN

Try oral steroids. Begin with prednisone, 20 - 40 mg PO Q day; attempt to taper prednisone after 5 - 7 days. Improved?

No
Yes → Physician–Nurse–Pharmacist consultation; consider lowest effective dose

Physician-Nurse-Pharmacist consultation. Would patient benefit from biliary stent?

Psychosocial Assessment and Intervention Guide

When the patient has been referred to the hospice program, a nurse and social worker visit is generated. These guidelines may be used to assess the patient.

Evaluate patient's support system:

- What support system is in place for the patient?
- Who are the key family members that have created positive and negative influences in the patient's life? Explore relationship with spouse or significant other, siblings, children, extended family.
- Who are the key non family members that play a role in support? Explore relationships with neighbors, co-workers, church, community.
- What is the available paid and unpaid support for the patient?
- Are any of these relationships at risk for present or future pathologic grief? Who will need referral to grief support services now and after patient's death? Consider referral through the hospice bereavement program or other community support services.
- Explore patient's hopes and plans for the next few days, weeks, months. Assist in setting realistic goals and implementing plans to achieve those goals.
- Would patient benefit from a hospice volunteer, a lifeline installation, or community service such as respite, chore, or copes worker? Assist with application if needed.
- Is patient and family receptive to placement in an adult family home, assisted living facility or nursing home, as appropriate, as patient declines? If so, identify preferences early; reviewing strengths and weaknesses of the different facilities.

Evaluate patient's educational history

- If patient unable to read or write, create a plan to assure proper understanding of teaching.
- For language barriers, assure presence of interpreter.
- For cultural barriers, see *Cultural Sensitivity Guidelines*.
- What are patient's hobbies or outside interests?
- Assist in adapting activities to patient's current level of activity and ability (e.g. talking books, assist devices in the home).

What are patient's financial resources?
- Are patient's current resources adequate to meet patient's definition of comfort?
- Is patient eligible for additional funding from other resources?
- Does a family member qualify to be paid as a chore worker?
- If so, assist with application process for accessing outside funds to state, federal or community programs; consider an application to decrease patient's cost of care.
- Does patient qualify for an indigent pharmaceutical program?

Assess patient's emotional state
- Assess quality of life as defined by the patient (Document *QOL Score*)
- What is patient's personal death awareness? Consider using a personal death awareness survey to guide discussion. (See *Appendix*)
- What is the patient's history of coping with stressors in life?
- What is patient's expectation of self now and in the immediate future? Are these expectations realistic?
- Is patient currently receiving psychiatric care?
- Is there a history of psychiatric illness? Would patient benefit from a mini mental status exam by the RN or a mental health referral?
- Is patient depressed or anxious? (See *Depression/Anxiety Algorithm*)
- Is there a history or current concern with substance abuse?
- What is patient's cognitive status? Address issues of impaired orientation, memory, thought process, judgement, attention, concentration with the family. Prepare family for potential need to access additional support in the home or transfer to long-term care facility as patient care needs escalate.
- Review expected trajectory of impairment of patient awareness with the death process.
- Discuss ways to compensate or adapt the environment to optimize patient care and communication, especially as visual, auditory, speech, oral intake and other physical abilities decline.

Continued on next page

- Explore patient's perception of self, relationship to others, and to God. (See *Spiritual Assessment Guideline*; refer to chaplain or spiritual supporter as appropriate)
- Identify spiritual affiliations in the community and request permission to inform of patient's involvement with the hospice team.
- Identify cultural heritages, beliefs, rituals, that facilitate comfort for the patient and family's preparation for death.
- What unfinished business is yet to be done? Assist with creating a living will and durable power of attorney for health care and for estate. Refer to appropriate legal counsel as needed.
- Assist with designation for mortuary services, planning for memorial services if requested. Identify prearrangements for funeral and disposition when deceased.
- Assist family with plans for closure. Would they benefit from creating scrapbooks, recording stories, songs, thoughts?

Establish plan of care

- Periodic reassessments to determine patient and family concerns, feelings, and fears.
- Assist with adaptation to patient's declining physical and emotional condition. Assist with the anticipatory grief process.
- Assess if additional support is needed. Assure community resources are in place.
- Periodic evaluation of special needs and patient/family's ability to comprehend teaching and education from the hospice team.

Secretions Assessment

Assessment Guidelines
- Assess ability to swallow and chew
- Assess for presence of oral Candida or mucositis
  (See *Oral Candidiasis Algorithm* or *Mucositis Algorithm*)
- Assess stage of disease using *ECOG Scale*
- Assess characteristics of secretions
- Assess oral hygiene practices
- Assess oral intake of fluids
- Review patient medication list for xerostomic (dry mouth) producing side effects
- Recent radiation or chemotherapy?
- Assess patient and family concerns regarding this symptom

Physician-Nurse-Pharmacist consultation for etiology not addressed in algorithm

Initiate *Secretions Algorithm* and/or proceed to associated algorithms

Implement appropriate non-pharmacologic interventions
(See *Secretions Treatment Algorithm*)

Secretion Treatment Algorithm is on the next two pages.

Non-Pharmacologic Interventions

Non-Pharmacologic interventions for xerostomia:
• Encourage frequent intake of oral fluids • Encourage good oral care • Avoid smoking, alcohol, caffeine and spicy foods • Use artificial saliva • Chew sugarless gum • Suck sugarless candy, especially citrus

Non-Pharmacologic interventions for increased secretions:
• Position patient to better deal with secretions • Suctioning • Absorbant towels to gather secretions

Secretions Treatment Algorithm

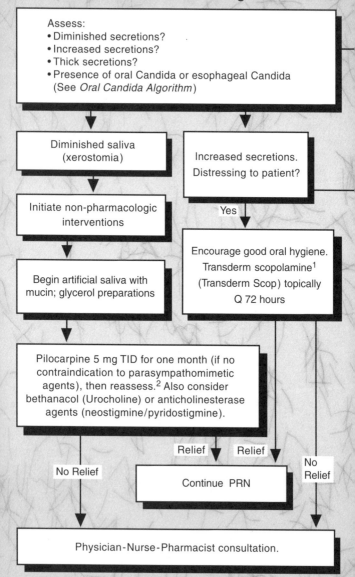

Assess:
- Diminished secretions?
- Increased secretions?
- Thick secretions?
- Presence of oral Candida or esophageal Candida (See *Oral Candida Algorithm*)

Diminished saliva (xerostomia)

Increased secretions. Distressing to patient?

Initiate non-pharmacologic interventions

Yes

Encourage good oral hygiene. Transderm scopolamine[1] (Transderm Scop) topically Q 72 hours

Begin artificial saliva with mucin; glycerol preparations

Pilocarpine 5 mg TID for one month (if no contraindication to parasympathomimetic agents), then reassess.[2] Also consider bethanacol (Urocholine) or anticholinesterase agents (neostigmine/pyridostigmine).

Relief   Relief

No Relief

Continue PRN

No Relief

Physician-Nurse-Pharmacist consultation.

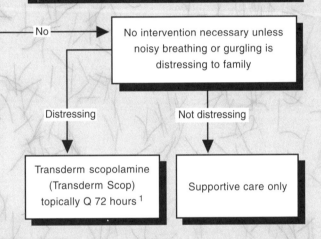

For thick secretions:
- Guaifenesin 10 - 20 mL (100 mg / 5 mL) PO Q 4 hours
- Potassium Iodide (PIMA) 5 - 10 mL PO TID [3]

If no relief, Physician-Nurse-Pharmacist consultation. Consider a trial of nebulized normal saline Q 4 hours PRN.

No → No intervention necessary unless noisy breathing or gurgling is distressing to family

Distressing

Not distressing

Transderm scopolamine (Transderm Scop) topically Q 72 hours [1]

Supportive care only

[1] Alternatives to scopolamine patches include scopolamine time released capsules or hyoscyamine preparations (Cystospaz-M, Levsinex Timecaps, Levsin drops)

[2] Avoid pilocarpine in patients with endstage cardiac, pulmonary, hepatic disease, or active ulcers.

[3] Avoid using PIMA in patients with hyperthyroidism and/ or renal disease

Seizure Assessment

- Assess for hypoglycemia
- If seizure is observed, is patient in a recovery position? (preferably on side)
- Assess airway (Does patient require jaw lift? Is suctioning needed?)
- If patient continues to seize without spontaneous termination, consider available routes of drug administration (intravenous, intramuscular, rectal administration) [See *Seizure Treatment Algorithm*]
- Are medications contributing to the seizure disorder? (i.e. oral hypoglycemic agents)
- Is an underlying medical condition causing the seizure or contributing to the seizure disorder? (hyponatremia, hypercalcemia, hypomagnesemia, hypotension, hypoxemia, withdrawal)
- Assess stage of disease using ECOG Scale (See *Appendix*)
- Assess seizure history (Is this a new onset seizure? What is the frequency of seizures?)
- Assess for injuries related to the seizure (intraoral abrasions or lacerations, musculoskeletal trauma)
- Assess current anti-seizure medications (What is the dosing of the current anti-seizure medications? Is the patient compliant with the dosing regimen? Is there a recent drug level (eg. phenytoin, phenobarbital, valproate or tegretol level)?
- Does the patient have known or suspected cerebral lesions? Does patient have a headache? Visual changes? Tinnitus?
- Assess for focal neurologic findings. Is there a history of stroke?
- Have seizure precautions been implemented? (padding and pillows, armrails to help keep patient in bed, no driving discussion)

Physician-Nurse-Pharmacist consultation for etiology not addressed in algorithm	Initiate *Seizure Algorithm* and/or proceed to associated algorithms	

Implement appropriate non-pharmacologic interventions (See *Seizure Algorithm*)

Seizure Assessment

Non-Pharmacologic Interventions

• Initiate general seizure precautions (padding, safe environment, no driving, calm soothing environment) • During seizure, if possible place patient on side • Jaw lift may sometimes be necessary to open and maintain airway after a seizure • Educate patient regarding avoidance of seizure stimulants (avoid alcohol and other substance abuse) • Do not put anything in patient's oral cavity • After seizure, consider suctioning patient if necessary to assist with oral secretions • Educate patient and caregivers regarding the seizure disorder and the expected post-ictal phase • After seizure, attend to any musculoskeletal injuries (ice, immobilization) • If hypotensive, patient should be supine; legs elevated • If patient is having a hypoglycemic seizure, administer oral glucose (juice, instant glucose, candy) if feasible • Patient and family education regarding treatment options, medications and anticipated effects

Footnotes (Refer to algorithm on the next page)
Seizure Treatment - Acutely seizing patient

1 When no intravenous access is available, alternatives to lorazepam include the following: **diazepam** 5 -10 mg IM, **diazepam** 10 mg PR (Consider **Diastat Rectal Gel**; alternatively **pentobarbital (Nembutal)** 60 mg PR).

2 Alternative therapy to phenytoin (Dilantin) is **fosphenytoin** (Cerebyx) 15 - 20 mg phenytoin equivalent/kg intravenous loading dose infused at 100 - 150 mg PE/minute. **Fosphenytoin** may also be given IM. The daily maintenance dose of **fosphenytoin** (Cerebyx) is 5 - 10 mg PE/kg intravenous at 150 mg PE/minute (PE=phenytoin equivalent)

3 **Midazolam** (Versed) given as a continuous infusion is usually adminstered 0.02 - 0.10 mg/kg/hr (1 - 7 mg/hr).

4 In the rare instance when **lidocaine 2%** is given to control seizures, lidocaine is administered 1.5 mg/kg IV or SC. When no intravenous access is available, **lidocaine 4%** may be administered intramuscular at a dose of 2 - 3 mg/kg.

5 **Etomidate** for seizure control is given intravenous 0.3 mg/kg, infused at 20 μg/kg/min. (May cause apnea.)

Seizure Treatment
Acutely Seizing Patient

Patient with seizure. Immediate pharmacotherapy may not be necessary for a seizure of short duration. Protracted seizures, in excess of 5 - 10 minutes often require interventions. Patients currently taking anticonvulsants should not receive the full loading doses of medications described below.

↓

Assess airway, breathing, circulation. Ensure adequate airway and oxygenation. Check blood pressure, pulse and temperature. Finger stick glucose to assess for hypoglycemia. Consider labs for metabolic screen (e.g. sodium and calcium)

↓

If hypoglycemic, correct hypoglycemia (therapeutic options: glucose containing candy, juice, instant oral glucose, intravenous glucose, and glucagon 1 mg IM, SC, IV)[1]

Is intravenous access available

No | Yes

Lorazepam (Ativan) 1 - 2 mg IV Q 3 - 4 min; maximum 30 mg

Seizure Continues

- Lorazepam 5 -10 mg IM
- Lorazepam 4 mg PR
  May repeat dose every 5 - 10 minutes if needed *

Phenytoin (Dilantin) 18 mg/kg intravenously over 30 minutes; the maximum rate of infusion is 50 mg/min. Monitor heart rate (bradycardia) and blood pressure (hypotension).[2]

Seizure Continues

Phenobarbital 20 mg/kg IV (maximum rate 100 mg/min)

Seizure Continues

Physician - Nurse - Pharmacist consultation; consider continuous IV or SC infusion of midazolam[3] (Versed), lidocaine[4] or etomidate[5]. (Apnea may occur.)

Proceed to *Seizure Control Therapies* when the acute seizure has been controlled

Seizure Treatment
Seizure Control Therapies

Physician - Nurse consultation prior to initiating chronic anticonvulsant therapy. Medications and therapies listed below are commonly used to control seizures; other regimens also exist. Maintenance therapy with anti-seizure medications may be neuroprotective in patients with known causes.

Address potentially treatable etiologies:

- Cerebral metastases - dexamethasone, radiation therapy, chemotherapy
- Hyponatremia - Fluid restriction, intravenous sodium chloride, medication adjustment (i.e. diuretics)
- Hypercalcemia - Encourage fluids
- Hypoglycemic reactions - Medication and dietary adjustments
- Hypoxemia - Supplemental oxygen
- Hypomagnesemia - Supplemental magnesium
- Substance abuse - Eliminate substance abuse, support withdrawal
- Infectious etiologies (meningitis, cerebral abscess, encephalitis) - Administer antibiotics according to the patient's directives

Grand Mal Seizure Medications

- Phenytoin (Dilantin) - Loading dose 15 -18 mg/kg. When given intravenously, the maximum rate of infusion is 50 mg/min; monitor blood pressure and heart rate for hypotension and bradycardia. Oral loading may be 300 mg PO every 2 - 3 hours for 3 doses. The usual adult daily dose is 300 mg/day.
- Phenobarbital - The loading dose is 20 mg/kg intravenously; maximum rate of infusion 100 mg/min. The usual adult daily dose is 60 -200 mg per day; doses are usually divided TID. Delivery may be orally or rectally.

Partial Seizures & Partial Complex Seizures

- Carbamazepine (Tegretol) - The initial adult dose is 200 mg PO BID; alternatively, 5 mL of suspension (100 mg/5 mL) QID. Doses are increased by 200 mg per day in divided doses. Maximum daily dose for an adult is 1.2 g/day.
- Ethosuximide (Zarontin) - The adult dose is 500 mg PO per day.
- Gabapentin (Neurontin) - For adults, initially give 300 mg PO HS on day 1, 300 mg PO BID on day 2, then 300 mg PO TID on day 3. Dosage increased as needed to 1,800 mg/day in divided doses.
- Valproic acid (Depakene) - The adult dose is 15 mg/kg PO daily, then increased by 5 to 10 mg/kg daily at weekly intervals up to a maximum of 60 mg/kg daily.

Skin Care Assessment

- Assess the patient's and caregiver's goals for skin care
- Assess patient and family's current knowledge regarding skin care
- Assess patient's activity level, mobility, and ability to ambulate
- Establish the need for a written plan for skin care
- Is the patient at high risk for ulcerations? Document patient's risk using the *Braden Scale*. (See *Braden Scale* page 110)
- Psychosocial assessment; review patient's and caregiver's motivation to follow plan of care. (See *Psychosocial Algorithm*)
- For any areas of skin breakdown, note location, dimensions, appearance of wound and edges, tenderness, drainage, status of surrounding skin, stage of ulcer, and odor (See *Pressure Ulcer Staging* in *Appendix*)
- Are there signs of skin infection? (redness, warmth, tenderness, swelling, purulent drainage, foul odor, fever, chills)
- Are there signs of skin ulceration, weeping, or dermatitis? (See *Skin Care Guidelines*)
- Assess positioning and use of cushions
- Assess for moisture or incontinence (See *Urinary Incontinence Algorithm* and *Diarrhea Algorithm*)
- Is the skin surrounding areas of ulceration protected?
- Are skin conditions currently being treated? If so, what products are being used?
- Assess patient transfer procedure (Are shearing forces produced?)
- Are restraints being used?
- Assess apparel, socks, and footware
- Are finger nails properly trimmed to minimize scratches?
- Assess ECOG for progression of disease state (See *Appendix* for functional performance scales)
- Assess current medications (Is an allergic reaction to a medication a possibility?)
- Assess the patient's ability to perceive pain, sensation, and and pressure
- Assess peripheral perfusion (quality of pulses, warmth, capillary refill, presence of hair)
- Assess nutritional and hydration status. Evaluate amount of fluid intake and output. Provide interventions appropriate to meet the hydration needs of the patient (See *Skin Care Guideline - Nutrition and Hydration*)

Adapted from Providence Central Washington Service Area Skin Care Guidelines

Skin Care Assessment

→ Initiate *Skin Care Treatment Algorithm* and/or
proceed to other associated algorithms

→ Implement appropriate
non-pharmacologic interventions

→ Physician–Nurse–Pharmacist
consultation for etiology not addressed in this algorithm

The Braden Scale is used as a risk assessment tool for pressure ulcers of the skin.

Low risk   15-16
Moderate risk   13-14
High risk   12 or less

Braden Scale for Assessing Pressure Ulcer Risk

	1. Completely limited	2. Very limited	3. Slightly limited	4. No impairment	Total
Sensory Perception — Ability to respond meaningfully to pressure related discomfort	Unresponsive (does not moan, flinch, or grasp) to painful stimuli, due to diminished level of consciousness or sedation OR limited ability to feel pain over most of body surface	Responds only to painful stimuli. Cannot communicate discomfort except by moaning or restlessness OR has a sensory impairment which limits the ability to feel pain or discomfort over half of the body	Responds to verbal commands but cannot always communicate discomfort or need to be turned OR has some sensory impairment which limits ability to feel pain or discomfort in 1 or 2 extremities		
Moisture — Degree to which skin is exposed to moisture	**1. Constantly moist:** Skin is kept moist almost constantly by perspiration, urine, etc. Dampness is detected every time patient is moved or turned	**2. Moist:** Skin is often but not always moist. Linen must be changed at least once a shift	**3. Occasionally moist:** Skin is occasionally moist, requiring an extra linen change approximately once a day	**4. Rarely moist** Skin is usually dry; linen requires changing only at routine intervals	
Activity — Degree of physical activity	**1. Bedfast:** Confined to bed	**2. Chairfast:** Ability to walk severely limited or nonexistent. Cannot bear own weight and/or must be assisted into chair or wheel chair	**3. Walks occasionally:** Walks occasionally during day but for very short distances, with or without assistance. Spends majority of each shift in bed or chair	**4. Walks frequently:** Walks outside the room at least twice a day and inside room at least once every 2 hours during waking hours	

	1. Completely immobile:	2. Very limited:	3. Slightly limited:	4. No limitations:
Mobility Ability to change and control body position	Does not make even slight changes in body or extremity position without assistance	Makes occasional slight changes in body or extremity position but unable to make frequent or significant changes independently	Makes frequent though slight changes in body or extremity position independently	Makes major and frequent changes in position without assistance
	1. Very poor:	**2. Probably inadequate:**	**3. Adequate:**	**4. Excellent:**
Nutrition Usual food intake pattern	Never eats a complete meal. Rarely eats more than 1/3 of any food offered. Eats 2 servings or less of protein (meat or dairy products)per day. Does not take a liquid dietary supplement, or is NPO[1] and/or maintained on clear liquids or IV[2] for more than 5 days	Rarely eats a complete meal and generally eats only about 1/2 of any food offered. Protein intake includes only 3 servings of meat or dairy products per day. Occasionally will take a dietary supplement, OR receives less than optimum amount of liquid diet or tube feeding	Eats over half of most meals. Eats a total of 4 servings of protein (meat, dairy products) each day. Occasionally will refuse a meal, but will usually take a supplement if offered, OR is on a tube feeding or TPN[3] regimen, which probably meets most of nutritional needs	Eats most of every meal. Never refuses a meal. Usually eats a total of 4 or more servings of meat and dairy products. Occasionally eats between meals. Does not require supplementation
	1. Problem	**2. Potential problem**	**3. No apparent problem**	
Friction/shear	Requires moderate to maximum assistance in moving. Complete lifting without sliding against sheets is impossible. Frequent slides down in bed or chair, requiring frequent repositioning with maximum assistance. Spasticity, contractures, or agitation leads to almost constant friction	Moves feebly or requires minimum assistance. During a move skin probably slides to some extent against sheets, chair, restraints, or other devices. Maintains relatively good position in chair or bed most of the time but occasionally slides down	Moves in bed and in chair independently and has sufficient muscle strength to lift up completely during move. Maintains good position in bed or chair at all times	

[1]NPO-Nothing by mouth [2]IV-Intravenously [3]TPN-Total parenteral nutrition

(Source Barbara Braden and Nancy Bergstrom, 1988)

Skin Care Guidelines

For details see *Skin Care Guidelines* and *Dressing and Solution Information*. Also, see sections dealing with incontinence, arterial and venous stasis ulcer management.

General interventions
- Establish goals to maintain comfort and promote healing
- Establish good preventative skin care for high risk patients.
- Educate patient and caregiver regarding proper positioning, transferring, and turning techniques
- Educate patient and family regarding methods to prevent skin breakdown
- Develop a written plan for care that is available to the patient and caregivers. (Include the following: etiology and risk factors for pressure ulcers, proper skin assessment, individualized program for skin care, demonstration of positioning to decrease risk of tissue breakdown, and demonstration of assist devices.)
- Reposition patient every two hours
- Use pillows or foam wedges to keep bony prominences from direct contact
- Use pressure relieving devices on the heels (*Oscar Splint, Span-Aid boot/anklet*)
- Use lifting devices to move rather than drag patient
- Pressure-reducing mattress (*foam, static air, alternating air, gel, or water mattress*)
- Encourage patient to shift weight every 15 minutes
- Use pressure-reducing devices for seating surfaces (avoid donut-type devices)
- Avoid massage over bony prominences
- Use lubricants to reduce friction injuries
- Encourage prompt skin care at the time of soiling
- Minimize skin exposure to moisture; minimize use of products that hold moisture against skin (Chux, adult briefs)
- When moisture cannot be controlled, use "geri pad" or underpad; is patient a candidate for a catheter?
- Encourage nutrition and hydration support as indicated
- Avoid alcohol containing lotions
- Reduce use of restraints
- Attention to trimming nails to avoid scratches

Skin Care Guidelines

General interventions continued

- Encourage properly fitting apparel, socks, and footwear
- Maintain the head of the bed in the lowest possible position
- Assign caregiver to pressure ulcer prevention role
- Use powders for moist areas (under breast, groin, abdominal folds)
- Encourage proper bathing (avoid scalding water, gentle patting to dry skin)
- Mechanical debridement of skin ulcers includes the following therapies: scrubbing, whirlpool, wet to dry dressings, irrigation, showering
- Enzymatic debridement solution if indicated (See *Dressing and Solution Information*) Use daily; should not harm the peri-wound tissue
- Autolysis debridement (using the body's immune system) includes the following: topical dressings (*normal saline dressing*), transparent membrane (*Tegaderm*), hydrocolloid (*DuoDerm, Tegasorb, Restore*), polyurethane foams (*Epilock, Mitraflex*), foams (*PolyMem or PolyWic*) See *Dressings and Solution Information*
- Update plan every two weeks

Professor Bud's Skin Care

Mix equal parts of the following:
- 100% aloe vera gel
- Glycerin
- Bay rum
- Baby oil

Apply to dry areas liberally. Apply daily.

Developed by Bud Williams - a beloved hospice patient with ALS who brought the gift of laughter and cultivated the self-esteem of many of our community's children with Professor Bud's Mini-Circus.

Skin Care Guidelines

Dressing and solution information *

Dressings

- Traditional - normal saline with materials such as: *Gauze, NuGauze, Kerlix Fluffs, Sofwick*
- Transparent membranes - *Tegaderm*
- Polyurethane Foam - *Lyofoam, Epilock, Mitraflex*
- Foam - *PolyMem*
- Hydrogel - Keeps the wound bed moist and provides a healing environment. *Curasol Gel Wound Dressing (HealthPoint), Carrasyn Dermal Wound Gel*
- Hydrocolloid - *Comfeel, Duoderm, Tegasorb, Restore*
- Calcium Alginate - Use with moderate to heavy exudative wounds. *Kaltostat, Sorbsan, Algiderm*
- Hydrofiber Dressing - Use with moderate to heavy exudative wounds. *Aquacel (ConvaTec)*
- Wound Filler - Use with moderate to heavy exudative wounds *Poly Wic*

Enzymatic debridement - *Travase, Santyl, Elase, Panofil, Accuzyme*
   Avoid use to minimize tissue damage except in case of infected tissue

Solutions

- Traditional - normal saline
- Non toxic solutions (*Shurclens*)
- Antiseptic solutions
  - Acetic Acid - Effective against Pseudomonas Aeruginosa in superficial wounds
  - Hydrogen peroxide - Provides mechanical cleansing and some debridement by effervescent action
  - Sodium Hypochlorite - *Dakin's Solution, Chlorpactin* Effective against Staphylococcus, Streptococcus; controls odor
  - Metronidazole paste (create by crushing 1 gram tablets) for infected malodorous wounds
  - Povidone-Iodine - Broad-spectrum effectiveness when used on intact skin or small relatively clean wounds

Bleeding wounds

- *SurgiCel* or *Gelfoam* as indicated

---

* This list is not meant to be complete or to promote any given product. Products listed reflect Central Washington Providence Service area utilization at time of publication. A special thanks to Chris Ivy, NP.

Skin Care Guidelines

Document risk by using the Braden Scale

Preventative measures

- Daily personal care/hygiene routines
- Daily mobility/activity routines
- Skin protection with proper fitting apparel
- Prevent friction injuries - use transparent membranes (eg.*Tegaderm*) and hydrocolloid (e.g. *Duoderm, Comfeel*)
- Provide skin protective barriers with paste, creams, ointments
- Apply liberally; no need to remove all of the topical skin protective barrier each time
- Mineral oil makes removal easier
- Be aware that protective barriers may potentiate fungal or yeast infections
- Examples: *Baza, Destine, Calmoseptine, zinc oxide*
- Personal safety (bed rails, layout of room, lights, etc.)
- Important to teach patient and caregiver how to examine the skin especially over bony prominences and to recognize the signs of a developing pressure ulcer
- Important to teach patient and caregiver how to do pressure releases, turn and position frequently, and educate on specific preventive measures as listed below

Infection control & wound care

- Irrigation or showering are the easiest cleansing technique
- Use appropriate solutions: normal saline, nontoxic solutions (e.g. *ShurClens*) or antiseptics
- Air dry wounds, if appropriate; never use hair dryers or direct heat lamps
- Apply appropriate dressings

Primary dressings: wound packing products and listed trade name examples

- Traditional: *NuGauze strips, Kerlix fluff or roll, gauze*
- Hydrogels: *Carrasyn dermal wound gel, Duoderm gel, Scott normal gel*
- Calcium alginate * : *Sorbsan, Algiderm, Kaltostat*
  *If a calcium alginate dressing sticks to wound bed, the wound is too dry to be using this product
- Wound filler: *PolyWic*

Skin Care Guidelines continued

Secondary dressings:
- Traditional: *gauze, Kerlix fluff/ABD*
- Hydrocolloid: *DuoDerm, Comfeel, Tegasorb, Restore* (not for Stage 3 ulcers)
- Polyurethane foam: *Lyofoam, Epilock, Mitraflex*
- Foam: *PolyMem*
- Antibiotic paste (e.g. *crushed metronidazole tablets -Flagyl*) for infected, malodorous wounds
- Consult plastic surgeon for complex wound care requiring operating room debridement or skin grafts/flaps

Preservation of circulation
- Keep body and room temperature warm to facilitate normal skin temperature
- Is patient a candidate for antiplatelet or viscosity lowering agent?

Nutrition and hydration
- Attention to nutrition & hydration sufficient to maintain healing environment/skin integrity
- Establish patient and caregiver's goals of therapy; is an advanced directive in place?
- Calculate caloric needs of patient to optimize healing
- Guidelines for optimal healing for pressure ulcers

  Calories required - 30 to 35 calories/kg/day
  Supplements - Several protein shakes/day
  Grams of protein - 1.25 to 1.50 grams of protein/kg/day
  Fluids - normal 2000-3000 mL/day;
  Urine output > 20 mL/hour, light straw color and no odor
- Adapt nutrition and hydration for complex cardiac, pulmonary, renal, or severe end stage patients
- Vitamins & minerals supplement - Multi or prenatal vitamin pill daily
- Blood Glucose level of > 200 mg/dL may increase risk for infection and delay healing
- Monitor fluid intake and output; counsel on methods to optimize hydration status
- Document interval weights
- Review current medications, including herbal, mineral and vitamin supplements
- Consider registered dietician consultation

Skin Care Guidelines

Skin Care Guidelines continued

Pressure relief for skin

- Attention to pressure prone areas of the body and implement reduction/relief measures
- Implement a regular turning and positioning schedule
- Consider designating one responsible caregiver to oversee its implementation
- Limit time on involved site especially in patient with multiple ulcers
- Decrease use of equipment that may increase the risk of pressure ulcers:
  - Wheel chairs may cause pressure ulcers if the bottom has a sling effect
  - Old non-supportive mattresses *
  - Lounge chairs: positioning may potentiate focal pressure to sacrococcygeal area
  - Sliding boards
- Utilize pressure reduction aids; categorical examples listed below
  - Heel protectors (*Oscar splint; Span Aid boot/anklet*)
  - 4-6 inch high density foam wheelchair cushions (*SpanAid*) or mattresses (*High-Float, Geo Matt*)
  - Lateral rotation air flow mattress (*Micro 2*) or air flow mattress overlay (*FirstStep by KCI or Flexicair by Hill Rhon*)
  - Low air loss specialty bed (*Kinaire by KCI; Flexicair by Hill Rhon*)
  - Water and gel mattresses (*RIK Fluid Mattress*)

* Eggcrate mattresses are good for comfort. Eggcrates are best applied to a supportive mattress; they do nothing to reduce pressure on the body and should not be used if a patient has a decubitus ulceration.

Pain management

- Assess pain (See *Pain Management Algorithms* appropriate to severity of pain and current medications)
- Decrease pain by incorporating pain medications, positioning, and frequency of care required; treat infections if indicated.
- For neuropathic pain, see *Adjuvant Medication Guide Neuropathic pain in Appendix*
- Be aware of impaired sensation, especially in patients with chronic small vessel disease

Skin Care Guidelines continued

Multidisciplinary services

- Consult palliative medicine/hospice specialist, if appropriate
- Consult orthopedist, physiatrist, or physical therapist, as indicated
  - May maximize mobility/activity; safe transfers
  - Range of motion exercises to maintain function
- Consult occupational therapist, as indicated - Aid in evaluating sitting surfaces, need for therapeutic support surfaces, splints, and braces
- Consult podiatrist for foot care
- Consult plastic surgeon, as indicated, for complex wound care
- Consult mental health professionals as indicated (See *Anxiety* and *Depression Treatment Algorithms*)
- Consult complementary medicine providers such as masseurs, accupuncturists, herbalists, energy work therapists, etc., as indicated

Skin Care Guidelines

Skin Care Guidelines continued

Incontinence/Perineal skin management
(See *Urinary Incontinence Algorithm*)
- Cleanse well after each urination or defecation
  - May use soap and water, rinse well
  - Cleanse perineal skin with cleanser *Peri Wash II, Healthpoint Incontinent cleaner*; if cleanser burns use normal saline or soap and water; do not to scrub the involved area.
- Blot dry - Intrabuttock, perineum, areas under folds must be dried thoroughly to prevent skin breakdown and fungal infections
- Apply coat of skin protective barrier cream or ointment to entire perineal area
- Skin protection that may prevent skin breakdown
  - Prevents friction injuries
    - Transparent membrane: *Tegaderm*
    - Hydrocolloid: *DuoDerm, Comfeel*
  - Skin protective barriers paste/cream/ointment
    e.g. *Baza, Desitin, Calmoseptine*, zinc oxide
    Apply liberal amounts. No need to remove all of the topical skin protective barrier each time; mineral oil will make removal easier. Skin protective barriers may potentiate a fungal or yeast infection.
  - Goal is to cleanse and dry the skin as soon as soiled
- Managing incontinence
  - External devices
    Male external catheter - *Mentor External Catheter, Texas Catheter, Retracted Penis Pouch (Hollister), VP external balloon catheter*, 2 piece urostomy appliance, Male drip collectors, Female external urine appliance (*Hollister*)
    Stool collector-Fecal Incontinence Pouches (*ConvaTec/Hollister*)
  - Internal device
    Foley catheter may be option in severe cases; this may increase risk for urinary tract infection. See *Bladder Spasm Algorithm* for urinary tract infection suppressive therapy.
- Bedbound patients can use washable underpants or "geri pads". Avoid underwear/briefs except when the patient is up in the chair or ambulating.
- Turn frequently to increase circulation to the skin breakdown (See *Skin Care Guidelines - Preventative measures* also see *arterial and venous stasis ulcer* section if indicated)

Skin Care Guidelines continued

Arterial Ulcers and Diabetic Ulcers
- Cleansing protocol
  - Optimize pain management (See *Pain Algorithms*)
  - Initially irrigate with normal saline or nontoxic solution
    (See *Dressing and Solution Information Chart*)
  - Blot dry
- Topical Therapy - Goal is to prevent infection
  - Caution when there is cellulitis
    (See *Skin Care Treatment Algorithm*)
  - A topical antibiotic agent may be indicated
  - A systemic oral antibiotic may be required; control of
    infection aids in pain control
  - Betadine, Silvadene or other antimicrobial agents may
    be ordered
    (See *Dressing and Solution Information Chart*)
  - Moist wound healing is contraindicated over ischemic
    wounds unless surgery has been performed to restore
    perfusion; avoid occlusive dressings with arterial ulcers
    or with cellulitis.
  - Patients with altered immune systems need special
    attention; they will have impaired inflammatory responses
    and are at higher risk of infection.
  - Arterial ulcers may also be associated with osteomyelitis
- Appropriate dressings
  (See *Dressing and Solution Information Chart*)
  - Primary dressing - Wound packing products
    - Traditional: *NuGauze strips, gauze, Kerlix fluff or roll*
    - Hydrogel: *Carrasyn Dermal Wound Gel, DuoDerm Gel*
    - Calcium Alginate: *Sorbsan, Algiderm, Kaltostat*
      (If the dressing sticks to the wound bed, the wound is
      too dry to be using calcium alginate)
    - Wound Filler: *PolyWic*
  - Secondary dressing
    - Traditional: *Gauze, Kerlix fluff/ABD*
    - Hydrocolloid: *DuoDerm, Restore*
    - Polyurethane Foam: *Lyofoam, Epilock*
    - Foam: *PolyMem*

Skin Care Guidelines continued

Venous Stasis Ulcer (Venous Insufficiency Ulcer)

- Cleansing protocol
  - Optimize pain management (See *Pain Algorithms*)
  - Initially cleanse with normal saline or nontoxic solution (*ShurClens*)
  - Utilize gentle scrubbing technique, if tolerated
  - Rinse thoroughly with normal saline or nontoxic solution (*ShurClens*)
  - Ideally, allow to air dry 10-20 minutes; initially the ulcer site(s) will not dry, but will continue to have exudate

- Topical Therapy
  - Caution when there is cellulitis (See *Skin Care Treatment Algorithm*)
  - A topical antibacterial cream (not ointment)
  - Systemic or oral antibiotics may be required
  - Infection control minimizes pain
  - Avoid occlusive therapy on client's with cellulitis
  - Topical products to manage exudate (See *Dressing and Solution Information Chart*)
    - Hydrocolloid: *DuoDerm, Restore , Comfeel Contour Dressing, Comfeel Pressure Relief Dressing* (*Colorplast*)
    - Polyurethane Foam: *Lyofoam* (*Acme United Corporation*), *Epilock (CalgonVestal)*
    - Foam: *PolyMem*
    - Wound Filler: *PolyWic*
    - Calcium Alginate: *Sorbsan, Algiderm, Kaltostat* (If the dressing sticks to the wound bed, the wound is too dry to be using a calcium alginate)
    - Combination dressings: Collagen + calcium alginate
    - Traditional dressings (*Normal saline, gauze, Telfa, ABD*)
    - The frequency of dressing changes will be dictated by the amount of exudate

Skin Care Treatment Algorithm

If possible, determine the cause of the skin problem
(See *Skin Care Non-Pharmacologic Interventions*)

↓

For symptoms of pruritus, see *Pruritus Algorithm*

↓

For skin ulceration, see *Skin Care Guidelines;* see *Pressure Ulcer Staging Guide* in *Appendix*

↓

For allergic dermatitis/contact dermatitis, begin therapy with a topical steroid medication. Begin with 1.0% hydrocortisone cream applied BID as needed. Increase the steroid potency as needed (See *Steroid Potency Chart* in the *Appendix*)

↓

For skin soilage and dermatitis related to incontinence, see *Skin Care Guidelines* and *special section on Incontinence*

↓

With signs and symptoms of infection (cellulitis of the skin, folliculitis, purulent ulcerations), begin oral antibiotic therapy; start with cephalexin 500 mg PO QID for ten days. Alternative therapy would be erythromycin 333 mg PO TID for ten days. If additional gram negative bacteria coverage is needed ciprofloxacin 500 mg PO BID for ten days can be initiated in addition to the cephalexin or erythromycin.

↓

For dry skin conditions, begin BID to TID therapy with a moisturizing lotion or ointment. Some options include: Lac Hydrin, Keri lotion, Professor Bud's Skin Gel (page 113), Vaseline Intensive Care

↓

Physician - Nurse - Pharmacist consultation to discuss alternative diagnoses and treatment options

Notes

Sleep Disturbance Assessment

Assessment Guidelines:
- Delineate the pattern of insomnia

  Trouble falling asleep, but no trouble staying asleep?

  No trouble falling asleep but awakening on and off throughout the night?

  Early morning awakening, unable to go back to sleep?
- Is loss of sleep accompanied by unrelieved distressing symptoms, especially pain?
- Assess usual sleep pattern
- Assess medications for side effects
- Assess for unmet spiritual or emotional needs such as fear and anxiety (See *Spiritual and Psychosocial Assessments*)
- Frequent napping during the day?
- Assess for use of stimulants (i.e. smoker, caffeine intake)
- Does this patient have a sleep ritual?
- Is sleep disturbance a manifestation of depression?
- Are there recent changes in the patient's home setting?
- Sundowner's syndrome with increased restlessness in the evening?
- Does the patient have sleep apnea?

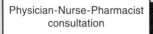

Physician-Nurse-Pharmacist consultation

Implement appropriate non-pharmacologic interventions

Initiate *Sleep Disturbance Algorithm* and/or proceed to other associated algorithms

Non-pharmacologic interventions

• Counsel patient on sleep hygiene practices • Eliminate stimulant intake • Discourage daytime napping • Increase daytime activities • Consult chaplain, social worker, volunteer coordinator to facilitate support for unmet emotional or spiritual needs • Pet therapy • Educate patient and family on treatment options, medications and anticipated effects

Sleep Disturbance Treatment Algorithm

Loss of sleep

Zolpidem (Ambien) 5 - 10 mg PO Q HS. Alternatively, temazepam (Restoril) 15 - 30 mg PO Q HS; caution in patients over 60 years old. If already on lorazepam (Ativan), consider doubling PRN nighttime dose.
Start low and go slow.

Relief

Continue PRN

No Relief after 3 days

Physician-Nurse-Pharmacist consultation. Consider starting antidepressants (See below). If patient is anxious, consider one time dose of lorazepam (Ativan) 2 mg PO or IM (See *Anxiety Treatment Algorithm*). If effective, use lorazepam as needed.

Sleep loss related to depression (See *Depression Algorithm*)

Trazodone (Desyrel) 25 mg PO QHS (range 25 - 100 mg PO HS). If ineffective Amitriptyline (Elavil) 10 - 25 mg, increase dose Q 3 days by 25 mg (maximum of 150 mg PO Q HS). Counsel on anticipated side effects.

Relief

No Relief

Continue PRN

Physician-Nurse-Pharmacist consultation. Consider use of selective serotonin release inhibitors* [fluoxetine (Prozac), paroxetine (Paxil), sertraline (Zoloft), venlafaxine (Effexor), citalopram (Celexa)]

* SSRI's are contraindicated in patients already taking MAO inhibitors; caution if already on a cyclic antidepressant.

Spiritual Assessment and Intervention Guide

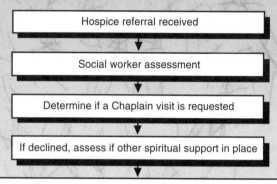

Hospice referral received

⬇

Social worker assessment

⬇

Determine if a Chaplain visit is requested

⬇

If declined, assess if other spiritual support in place

⬇

If other spiritual support is in place, request permission to notify key person of patient's enrollment in the hospice program and request their input into the process.

⬇

If declined, send spiritual care letter to patient and identified spiritual supporter; wait for patient or family to generate future request for additional support.

⬇

If the patient consents, proceed with Chaplain's visit, and spiritual assessment.

The spiritual assessment is divided into three categories or axes (vertical, horizontal and depth)

Spiritual Assessment
Vertical component (y axis):

What is patient's current perception of the image of God?
Are there past experiences that have contributed to this perception?
Does the patient read the Bible for comfort or support?
Explore these key concepts of the image of God:

- Is God a myth or real?
- Is God vengeful or loving?
- Is God passive or active in life?
- Is God distant or involved in day to day living?
- Is God forgiving or unforgiving?
- Is God spiteful or compassionate?
- Is God full of wrath or mercy?

Horizontal component (x axis):

What is the patient's perception of others?

Explore patient's experiences with forgiveness and lack of forgiveness.

Are interpersonal relationships a source of comfort or distress?

Encourage discussion of the meaning of these key relationships:

- Parents
- Siblings
- Children (or lack of children)
- Spouse or significant other
- Friends, coworkers, extended family
- Self (see below)
- God or other spiritual being (see above)

Depth component (z axis):

What is patient's perception of self?

Explore the emotional and spiritual components of death's meaning.

Does patient feel prepared for death? Are there issues of fear, joy, assurance of salvation, unfinished business?

Is patient accepting of the fact death is inevitable soon?

Consider using a personal death awareness inventory to guide discussion.

Tips on personal death awareness:

- Self is unconscious as well as conscious material
- Self awareness is adaptive
- Growth awareness will foster expansion of the consciousness into the formerly unconscious.
- Experiencing judgment from others may interfere with growth
- Suffering is often a natural component of growth
- Personal wholeness and acceptance is the goal

Establish plan of care   Also see Psychosocial Assessment Guidelines

- Encourage patient's personal story to be told with sharing or special aids such as scrapbooks; taping special thoughts, songs, stories; what is the patient's legacy?
- Are there inheritance issues patient wishes to address?
- Are plans for a funeral service made? Explore patient and family preferences.
- Identify who will sign the death certificate.
- Establish short, intermediate and long term goals with patient and caregivers.
- Reassess weekly patient's perception of goal fulfillment.
- Continue present plan or adapt as directed by patient and family.

Terminal Agitation Assessment

Assessment Guidelines:

- Assess for new, unrelieved or exacerbated pain (See *Pain Treatment Algorithm - Step 3*)
- Assess for hypoxia (See *Dyspnea Algorithm*)
- Assess bowel and bladder status - fecal impaction and/or bladder distension (See *Bowel and Bladder Algorithms*; see *Adjuvant Medication Guide*)
- Assess functional status using *ECOG Scale* or other scoring device (See *Appendix*)
- Assess for hallucinations, confusion, restlessness, muscle twitching, jerking and/or sweating
- Assess for unfinished business; consult social worker and/or chaplain (See *Psychosocial and Spiritual Assessment Guides*)
- Assess for spiritual distress; consult chaplain (See *Spiritual Algorithm*)
- Discuss with patient and caregivers the directive for comfort care and document the consensus directive
- Review *DNR* orders (*Do Not Resuscitate*) and counsel on potential for double effect (See *Ethical Decision Making Guidelines*)

Physician-Nurse-Pharmacist consultation prior to initiating *Terminal Agitation Algorithm*

Initiate non-pharmacologic interventions and provide support for both the patient and family

Initiate *Terminal Agitation Algorithm* and/or proceed to other associated algorithms

Non-Pharmacologic Interventions

• Subdued environment/reduce stimulus • Allow time for patient to talk freely about his/her concerns • Assess spiritual needs and intervene as needed • Softly lighted surroundings with familiar objects and familiar faces • Conversation with the patient and family should be calm and reassuring • Offer relaxation tapes • Relaxation/visualization/distraction therapy • Massage therapy • Aromatherapy • Therapeutic touch • Pet therapy • Patient and family education regarding treatment options, medications and anticipated effects

Terminal Agitation Treatment Algorithm

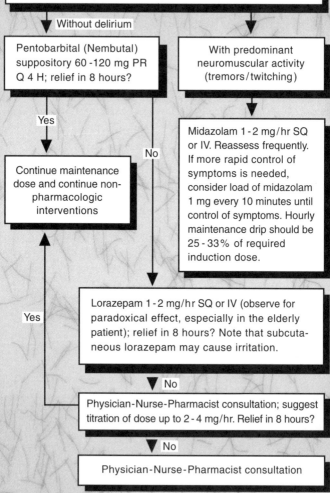

Severe restlessness or agitation. Physician-Nurse-Pharmacist consultation prior to initiating algorithm.*
Document the patient's directive on terminal care.
Consult Adjuvant Medication Guide.

Without delirium

Pentobarbital (Nembutal) suppository 60-120 mg PR Q 4 H; relief in 8 hours?

With predominant neuromuscular activity (tremors/twitching)

Yes

No

Continue maintenance dose and continue non-pharmacologic interventions

Midazolam 1-2 mg/hr SQ or IV. Reassess frequently. If more rapid control of symptoms is needed, consider load of midazolam 1 mg every 10 minutes until control of symptoms. Hourly maintenance drip should be 25-33% of required induction dose.

Yes

Lorazepam 1-2 mg/hr SQ or IV (observe for paradoxical effect, especially in the elderly patient); relief in 8 hours? Note that subcutaneous lorazepam may cause irritation.

No

Physician-Nurse-Pharmacist consultation; suggest titration of dose up to 2-4 mg/hr. Relief in 8 hours?

No

Physician-Nurse-Pharmacist consultation

* When the medical history and the physical examination suggest agitation that is compounded by alcohol or nicotine withdrawal, Physician-Nurse-Pharmacist consultation to discuss management (nicotine patch, alcohol withdrawal protocol)

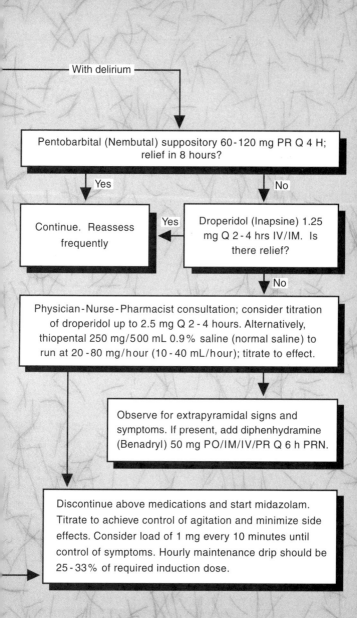

With delirium

Pentobarbital (Nembutal) suppository 60-120 mg PR Q 4 H; relief in 8 hours?

Yes → Continue. Reassess frequently

No → Droperidol (Inapsine) 1.25 mg Q 2-4 hrs IV/IM. Is there relief?

Yes → Continue. Reassess frequently

No → Physician-Nurse-Pharmacist consultation; consider titration of droperidol up to 2.5 mg Q 2-4 hours. Alternatively, thiopental 250 mg/500 mL 0.9% saline (normal saline) to run at 20-80 mg/hour (10-40 mL/hour); titrate to effect.

Observe for extrapyramidal signs and symptoms. If present, add diphenhydramine (Benadryl) 50 mg PO/IM/IV/PR Q 6 h PRN.

Discontinue above medications and start midazolam. Titrate to achieve control of agitation and minimize side effects. Consider load of 1 mg every 10 minutes until control of symptoms. Hourly maintenance drip should be 25-33% of required induction dose.

Appendix

Appendix Contents

Adjuvant Medication Chart

- Adjuvants and other medications are meant to augment, not be a substitute, for adequate doses of analgesics.

- The use of adjuvant medications may lead to the reduction in the amount of opioid medication needed.

- Aggressive titration of analgesics to control pain comes first.

- Refer to the specific treatment algorithm prior to initiating an adjuvant listed below for a particular symptom.

- Note that many of the adjuvants listed reflect the experience of practitioners in the field of hospice and palliative medicine; clinical trials are ongoing to validate their efficacy.

- Multipurpose, nonspecific adjuvants such as cyclic antidepressants, corticosteroids, clonidine, and neuroleptics have been shown to be efficacious often in uncontrolled clinical trials.

Major classes of adjuvant analgesics
Antidepressants
Alpha-2 adrenergic agonists
Anticonvulsants
Anesthetics (topical, subcutaneous, intravenous)
Anxiolytics
Corticosteroids
Gamma aminobutyric acid agonists
Muscle relaxants
N-methyl-D-aspartate receptor blockers
Neuroleptics
Osteoclast inhibitors
Psychostimulants
Radioactive nucleotide therapy
Sympatholytics

Adjuvant Medication Chart

Helpful drugs	Initial dose
Nociceptive pain Pain perceived to be secondary to somatic or visceral tissue damage perpetuating primary afferent nerve stimulation; goal of adjuvants often are to block noxious chemical mediators felt to activate or sensitize the nociceptors or act centrally to modulate the painful stimuli	
Somatic - Bone pain	
NSAIDS	(See NSAID formulary in Appendix)
Dexamethasone (Decadron)	• High dose regimens for acute painful syndrome or nerve compression: 100 mg IV followed by 20 mg IV QID and tapered over the subsequent weeks to control symptoms and reduce side effects • Low dose regimen: 4 - 8 mg PO TID, taper to effective dose • See Decadron suppository compounding in Appendix • Ineffective doses should always be tapered and discontinued • Equivalent steroid dose is 0.75 mg
Prednisone	• Equivalent steroid dose is 5 mg
Methylprednisolone	• Equivalent steroid dose is 4 mg
Refractory bone pain **Osteoclast inhibitors:**	
Calcitonin	100 - 200 IU IM QD x 7 day trial; continue if efficacious; intranasal 200 IU/spray/day is available
Biphosphonates: Pamidronate Clodronate* Sodium etidronate* Alendronate*	90 mg infusion Q 4 weeks
*Prophylactic benefits of these in metastatic disease is suggested; use in palliative medicine should be based on the patient's ECOG score and extent of disease	
Gallium nitrate	(current experience is limited)

Adjuvant Medication Chart

Helpful drugs	Initial dose
Radionucleotides Indications: • confirmed osteoblastic activity by bone scan • adequate bone marrow reserve documented with >60 K platelet count and WBC >2400 • given the 4-6 week delay in benefit, should only be considered in patients with a life expectancy of > 3 months Strontium - 89 Rhenium - 186 Samarium - 153	
L - Dopa	200 mg Q 6 - 8 hr (anecdotal reports only)
Muscle relaxants Baclofen (Lioresal)	5 mg PO TID, titrate to effect; MDD 90 mg / day; always taper off if ineffective
Diazepam (Valium)	2 - 5 mg PO TID, titrate to effect; also available in a rectal gel (Diastat) or suppository form
Although clinical data is lacking on the true relief of skeletal muscle spasm, the below medications reportedly are an option to NSAIDS, aspirin or acetaminophen to relieve muscle spasm	
Carisprodol (Soma)	350 - 700 mg QID
Methocarbamol (Robaxin)	1.5 grams QID
Chlorzoxazone (Parfon Forte)	250 - 750 mg PO QID
Cyclobenzaprine (Flexeril)	10-20 mg PO TID; use PRN or 3 week maximum continuous
Orphenadrine (Norflex)	100 mg PO BID
Visceral Dexamethasone (Decadron)	See above dosages; consider 10 mg IV trial, if line available, then oral or rectal dose regimens
Anticholinergics For visceral pain thought to be secondary to increased GI secretions or terminal bowel obstruction, consider: Hyoscyamine (Levsin solution- 0.125 mg/mL)	1 mL PO AC and Q HS
Glycopyrrolate (Robinul)	1 mg PO QD
Octreotide (Sandostatin) • somatostatin analog	25 - 50 µg SC QD, titrate up every few days based on patient response; goal is to achieve patient comfort by minimizing GI secretions and visceral distension

Adjuvant Medication Chart

Helpful drugs	Initial dose
Neuropathic pain with continuous dysesthesias	
First line therapy for patients who have not responded to an opioid	
Antidepressants (See Depression Algorithm)	
• Typical dosages for pain start low and titrate up every few days; dosages beyond standard antidepressant dosages are not likely to yield benefit	
• Go slow and assess impact; there is anecdotal experience noting that there may be a window of efficacy; to titrate dosages beyond this dose may lead to loss of analgesic efficacy	
• Patients responding to the TCA's may benefit from serum monitoring; this detects nonadherence to the medication scheduling or high metabolizers who may benefit from increased dosages	
Tricyclic antidepressants	
Amitriptyline (Elavil)	25 mg PO Q HS
Doxepin (Sinequan)	50 mg PO Q HS
Imipramine (Tofranil)	10 - 25 PO mg/day
Desipramine (Norpramin)	10 - 25 PO mg/day
Nortriptyline (Pamelor)	10 - 25 PO mg/day
Clomipramine (Anafranil)	25 mg PO QD
Non-tricyclic antidepressants See Depression algorithm for other SSRI's	
Paroxetine (Paxil)	10 mg PO QD (MDD 60 mg/day)
Trazodone (Desyrel)	50 mg PO QHS (MDD 600 mg/day)
Maprotiline (Ludiomil)	25 mg PO QHS (MDD 225 mg/day)
Anesthetics Contraindicated in patients with known compromised cardiac status	
Oral	
Mexiletine (Mexitil)	150 mg PO QD with food (MDD 1200 mg/day)
Tocainide (Tonocard)	400 mg PO QD, titrate up if effective (MDD 2400 mg/day)
IV or SC (anesthetic for crescendo neuropathic pain)	
Lidocaine	1 - 3 mg/kg infusion over 30 minutes then 1 - 3 mg/kg/h

Adjuvant Medication Chart

Helpful drugs	Initial dose
Refractory cases	For refractory pain, consider consultation with a pain or palliative care specialist.
Alpha-2 adrenergic agonists	
Clonidine (Catapres)	0.1 mg QD or 0.1 mg transdermal patch Q week
Anticonvulsants	
Gabapentin (Neurontin)	300 mg PO QD. Gradually titrate up; MDD 1800 mg (divided doses)
Carbamazepine (Tegretol)	200 mg PO Q 6 h
Phenytoin (Dilantin)	300 mg PO Q HS
Valproate (Depakene)	125 mg PO TID
Clonazepam (Klonopin)	0.5 mg PO QD; titrate up (MDD 20 mg)
Topical agents	
Capsaicin (Zostrix)	0.025 % cream applied QID to the affected area
Prilocaine 2.5%/lidocaine 2.5% cream (EMLA)	Apply 2.5 g of cream to intact skin requiring anesthetic. Cover site with occlusive dressing such as Tegaderm
Neuroleptics	
Prochlorperazine (Compazine)	10 mg PO QD (MDD 40 mg); RS 25 mg BID
Haloperidol (Haldol)	1 mg PO QD, titrate to effect (MDD 15 mg)
N-methyl-D-aspartate antagonists	
Dextromethorphan (Delsym)	60 mg PO TID (MDD 1000 g)
Ketamine (Ketalar)	0.1 mg/kg/hour infusions
Others	
Calcitonin	25 IU IM/day, titrate to relief, up to 100 - 200 IU IM/day; intranasal available 200 IU/spray/day
Baclofen (Lioresal)	5 mg PO TID, titrate to effect; MDD 90 mg; always taper off if ineffective

Adjuvant Medication Chart

Helpful drugs	Initial dose
Neuropathic pain with lancinating pain or paroxysmal dysesthesias	
Anticonvulsants First line therapy for patients not responding to an opioid alone	
Gabapentin (Neurontin)	300 mg PO QD. Gradually titrate to MDD 1800 mg (doses divided TID)
Carbamazepine (Tegretol)	200 mg PO Q 6 h
Phenytoin (Dilantin)	300 mg PO Q HS
Valproate (Depakene)	125 mg PO TID
Clonazepam (Klonopin)	0.5 mg PO QD; titrate up (MDD 20 mg)
Other Baclofen	5 mg PO TID, titrate to effect; (MDD 90 mg) Always taper off if ineffective
Refractory cases **Anesthetics** These medications should be used with caution in patients with known compromised cardiac status.	
Mexiletine (Mexitil)	150 mg PO QD with food (MDD 1200 mg/day)
Tocainide (Tonocard)	400 mg PO QD, titrate up if effective, (MDD 2400 mg/day)
Lidocaine (IV or SC)	1-3 mg/kg infusion over 30 minutes then 1-3 mg/kg/h
Tricyclic antidepressants	
Amitriptyline (Elavil)	25 mg PO Q HS
Doxepin (Sinequan)	50 mg PO Q HS
Imipramine (Tofranil)	10-25 PO mg/day
Desipramine (Norpramin)	10-25 PO mg/day
Nortriptyline (Pamelor)	10-25 PO mg/day
Clomipramine (Anafranil)	25 mg PO QD
Non-tricyclic antidepressants See Depression Algorithm for other SSRI's	
Paroxetine (Paxil)	10 mg PO QD (MDD 60 mg/day)
Trazodone (Desyrel)	50 mg PO QHS (MDD 600 mg/day)
Maprotiline (Ludiomil)	25 mg PO QHS (MDD 225 mg/day)
Neuroleptics	
Pimozide (Orap)	1 mg PO QD; titrate to effect (MDD 16 mg)
Methotrimeprazine	5 mg SC infusion titrate up to 80 mg
Fluphenazine (Prolixin deconate)	12.5 mg SC/IM Q 3 weeks

Adjuvant Medication Chart

Helpful drugs	Initial dose
Neuropathic pain with lancinating pain or paroxysmal dysesthesias (continued)	
Alpha-2 adrenergic agonists	
Clonidine (Catapres)	0.1 mg QD or 0.1 mg transdermal patch Q week
Topical agents	
Capsaicin (Zostrix)	0.025% cream applied QID to the affected area
Prilocaine 2.5%/lidocaine 2.5% cream (EMLA)	Apply 2.5 g of cream to intact skin requiring anesthetic. Cover site with occlusive dressing such as Tegaderm
N-methyl-D-aspartate antagonists	
Dextromethorphan (Delsym)	60 mg PO TID (MDD 1000 g)
Ketamine (Ketalar)	0.1 mg/kg/hour infusions
Other	
Calcitonin	25 IU IM/day, titrate to relief, up to 100-200 IU IM/day; intranasal available 200 IU/spray/day

Sympathetically maintained pain

- Thought to be stimulated efferent neurons in the sympathetic nervous system
- Clinical syndromes: reflex sympathetic dystrophy; causalgia
- Characterized by focal autonomic dysregulation (eg. swelling, sweating, vasomotor symptoms, tremors, dystonia; atrophic skin, nail, and hair regions; osteoporosis in region of pain)
- Phentolamine infusions are reportedly useful diagnostic tools
- Nerve blocks are the first line therapy; if blocks fail or are contraindicated, use above multipurpose adjuvants and neuropathic pain adjuvants

Dexamethasone (Decadron)	8 mg PO TID, taper to effect
Phenoxybenzamine (Dibenzyline)	10 mg PO BID (MDD 120 mg)
Nifedipine (Procardia)	10 mg PO TID (MDD 80 mg)
Prazosin (Minipress)	1 mg PO TID (MDD 20 mg)
Guanethidine (Ismelin)	5 mg PO QD (MDD 50 mg/day)
Nimodipine (Nimotop)	30 mg PO QD (MDD 360 mg/day)
Lidocaine IV or SC	1-3 mg/kg infusion over 30 minutes then 1-3 mg/kg/hr

Adjuvant Medication Chart

Helpful drugs	Initial dose
Affective/Idiopathic pain • See Agitation, Anxiety, Depression and Terminal Agitation Algorithms	
• Agitation/anxiety	
Lorazepam (Ativan) <small>Shorter dosing intervals may be needed; see Suppository recipes in the Appendix.</small>	0.5 - 2.0 mg PO/IM/SC Q 4 h
Haloperidol lactate (Haldol) <small>Observe pt for paradoxical effect of drug. (ie patient becoming more agitated inspite of medication)</small>	0.5 - 5 mg PO or IM; titrate up <small>Titrate up by 0.5 mg q 4 h until desired effect achieved; MDD=30 mg/day (Some patients may require up to 100 mg/day)</small>
Haloperidol decanoate	Dose is usually 10 - 15 times the oral dose, given IM Q 3 weeks
• Agitation/depression Consider cyclic antidepressant or SSRI. Consider use of a psychostimulant (See Opioid Induced Narcolepsy Algorithm)	
• Agitation/psychosis Haloperidol (Haldol) See above <small>Titrate upwards as needed to control symptoms. Observe pt for paradoxical effect of drug. (ie patient becoming more agitated inspite of medication)</small>	0.5 - 5 mg PO; 5 - 20 mg IM
• Agitation/terminal	
Pentobarbital (Nembutal)	30 - 100 mg PO; 60 - 200 mg PR Q 6 h
Midazolam (Versed)	0.4 mg - 2 mg per hour by continuous infusion with individual variation in MDD. Titrate until the patient is asleep and/or calmer.

Iatrogenic	
• Opioid induced nausea	
Meclizine (Antivert)	25 mg PO Q 8 h PRN
Transderm scopolamine patch	Change patch every 72 °
Alternatives to scopolamine patches include scopolamine time released capsules or hyoscyamine preparations (Cystospaz-M, Levsinex Timecaps, Levsin drops)	
• Opioid induced narcolepsy (sedation) <small>(Give doses early in the day to avoid sleep disturbances)</small>	
Dextroamphetamine (Dexidrine)	2.5 -5 mg PO Q AM and midday (MDD 40 mg/day)
Methylphenidate (Ritalin)	2.5 -5 mg PO Q AM and midday (MDD 60 mg/day)
Pemoline (Cylert)	18.75 mg PO Q AM, titrate Q 7 days (MDD 112.5 mg)

Adjuvant Medication Chart

Helpful drugs	Initial dose
Iatrogenic (continued)	
Nausea and Vomiting	
See Nausea Algorithm. For compounding instructions, see *Suppositories* in Appendix.	
Prochlorperazine (Compazine)	5 - 10 mg Q 6 h PO 2.0 - 10 mg Q 4 h IV 5 - 25 mg Q 12 h PR
Metoclopramide (Reglan)	10 - 20 mg PO AC and QHS
DBR suppositories [Decadron 10 mg, Benadryl 25 mg, Reglan 10 mg]	Q 6 h PR and PRN
RDA suppositories [Reglan 50 mg, Decadron 10 mg, Ativan 2 mg]	Q 6 h PR and PRN
DBA suppositories [Decadron 10 mg, Benadryl 25 mg, Ativan 2 mg]	Q 6 h PR and PRN
Sleep Disturbance See *Depression Algorithm* and *Sleep Disturbance Algorithm*	
Amitriptyline (Elavil)	25 mg PO Q HS
Doxepin (Sinequan)	50 mg PO Q HS
Hydroxyzine (Vistaril)	50 - 100 mg PO Q HS
Trazodone (Desyrel)	25 - 100 mg PO Q HS
Pruritus See *Pruritus Algorithm* and *Skin Care Algorithm* • Consider advancing from low to medium to high potency steroid compounds (See *Topical Steroid Table* in appendix) • Implement non-pharmacologic interventions • Consider preservative free compounds	
Diphenhydramine (Benadryl)	25 - 50 mg PO Q 6 h
Hydroxyzine (Vistaril, Atarax)	25 mg PO Q 6 - 8 h
Cimetidine (Tagamet)	300 mg PO Q 6 h

Non-Opioid Analgesics (NSAIDs, Salicylates)

Chemical Class	Generic Name	Half-Life (hr)
Cycloxygenase II inhibitors	Celecoxib (Celebrex)	11
N-acetyl-P-aminophenol	Acetaminophen (Tylenol)	1 - 3
Salicylates	Aspirin (enteric coated)	3 - 12
	Diflunisal (Dolobid)	8 - 12
	Cholinemagnesium trisalicylate (Trilisate)	8 - 12
	Salsalate (Disalcid)	8 - 12
Propionic Acids	Ibuprofen (Motrin)	3 - 4
	Naproxen (Anaprox)	13
	Naproxen Sodium (Naprosyn)	13
	Fenoprofen (Nalfon)	2 - 3
	Ketoprofen (Orudis)	2 - 3
	Flurbiprofen (Ansaid)	5 - 6
	Oxaprozin (Daypro)	50
Acetic Acids	Indomethacin (Indocin)	4 - 5
	Tolmetin (Tolectin)	1
See comments on next page regarding intravenous dosing of ketorolac (Toradol)	Sulindac (Clinoril)	14
	Diclofenac (Voltaren)	2
	Ketorolac (Toradol)	4 - 7
	Etodolac (Lodine)	1 - 2

Dosing Schedule	Recommended Starting Dose (mg/day) Dosing for > 50 kg body wt	Maximum Recommended Dose (mg/day)
Q 12 - 24 h	100 mg PO Q 12 h	400
Q 4 h	650 mg PO Q 4 h	4000
Q 4 - 6 h	650 mg PO Q 4 h	6000
Q 12 h	1000 x 1 then 500 Q 8 h	1500
Q 12 h	1500 x 1 then 500 Q 8 h	4000
Q 12 h	1500 x 1 then 500 Q 12 h	4000
Q 4 - 8 h	1200	4200
Q 12 h	500	1000
Q 12 h	550	1100
Q 6 h	800	3200
Q 6 - 8 h	150	300
Q 8 - 12 h	100	300
Q 24 h	1200	1800
Q 8 - 12 h	75	200
Q 6 - 8 h	600	2000
Q 12 h	300	400
Q 6 h	75	200
Q 4 - 6 h	120	240
Q 6 - 8 h	600	1000

For patients less than 50 kg, adjust dosage according to the weight

Non-Opioid Analgesics (NSAIDs, Salicylates)

Chemical Class	Generic Name	Half- Life (hr)
Oxicam	Piroxicam (Feldene)	45
Fenamates	Mefenamic Acid (Ponstel)	2
	Meclofenamic Acid (Meclomen)	2 - 4

Comments:

Celecoxib (Celebrex) has greatly reduced GI toxicity in comparison to NSAIDS. No significant impact on platelet function is reported.

Aspirin may not be tolerated as well as some NSAIDs. The half-life of aspirin increases with dose. Enteric coated aspirin is also available.

Diflusinal (Dolobid) has less GI toxicity than aspirin.

Choline magnesium trisalicylate (Trilisate) & salsalate (Disalcid), unlike other NSAIDS, have minimal GI toxicity & no effect on platelet aggregation, despite potent antiinflammatory effects. May therefore be particularly useful in some patients.

Ibuprofen is available over the counter; suspension available by prescription only.

Naproxen (Anaprox) is available as a suspension. Some studies show greater efficacy of higher doses, specifically 1500mg/day, with little to no increase in adverse affects. Long term efficacy of the dose and safety in a medically ill population is unknown. It should be used cautiously in selected patients.

Naproxen Sodium (Naprosyn): Some studies show greater efficacy of higher doses, specifically 1650 mg/day with little to no increase in adverse effects; long term efficacy of this dose and safety in a medically ill population is unknown, however, and it should be used cautiously in selected patients.

Flurbiprofen (Ansaid): Experience too limited to evaluate higher doses than those listed in the table, though it is likely that some patients would benefit from higher doses.

Dosing Schedule	Recommended Starting Dose (mg/day) Dosing for >50 kg body wt	Maximum Recommended Dose (mg/day)
q 24 h	20	40
q 6 h	500 x 1 then 250 mg q 6 h	1000
q 6 - 8 h	250	400

Indomethacin (Indocin) is available in sustained-release suspension and rectal formulations. Higher incidence of side effects, particularly GI and CNS, than propionic acids.

Sulindac (Clinoril) has less renal toxicity than other NSAIDs.

Diclofenac (Voltaren): Experience is too limited to evaluate higher doses than those listed in the table, though it is likely that some patients would benefit from higher doses.

Ketorolac (Toradol): Parenteral formulation available. When administering IV, use 30 mg dose. IM dose is 60 mg. Both efficacy and safety of long term administration remains to be determined. The current recommendation is to limit use to 5 days or less.

Piroxicam (Feldene): Administration of 40 mg for over 3 weeks is associated with a high incidence of peptic ulcer, especially in the elderly.

Mefenamic Acid (Ponstel): Not recommended for longer than one week and therefore not indicated in chronic pain therapy.

Although clinical experience suggests that any of the NSAIDs may be analgesic, pain is an approved indication only for diflunisal, ibuprofen, naproxen, naproxen sodium, fenoprofen, ketorolac .

For all non steroidal agents, at high doses stool should be checked for blood every 2 weeks and liver function tests, BUN and creatinine assessments, and urinalysis should be performed every 1-2 months.

Topical Steroid Potency Ranking

Group I is the super-potent category descending to Group VII which is the least potent. In general, there is no significant difference between agents within each group. However, within group I, Temovate cream and ointment are more potent.

Group	Brand Name	Generic Name
I	Temovate cream 0.05%	Clobetasol proprionate
	Temovate ointment 0.05%	
	Diprolene ointment 0.05%	Augmented betamethasone diproprionate
	Diprolene AF cream 0.05%	
	Psorcon ointment 0.05%	Diflorasone diacetate
	Ultravate cream 0.05%	Halobetasol proprionate
	Ultravate ointment 0.05%	
II	Cyclocort ointment 0.1%	Amcinonide
	Diprosone ointment 0.05%	Betamethasone diproprionate
	Elocone ointment 0.1%	Mometasone furoate
	Florone ointment 0.05%	Diflorisone diacetate
	Halog cream 0.1%	Halcinonide
	Halog ointment 0.1%	
	Halog solution 0.1%	
	Lidex cream 0.05%	Fluocinonide
	Lidex gel 0.05%	
	Lidex ointment 0.05%	
	Lidex solution 0.05%	
	Maxiflor gel/ointment 0.05%	Diflorasone diacetate
	Maxivate cream 0.05%	Betamethasone diproprionate
	Maxivate ointment 0.05%	
	Topicort cream 0.25%	Desoximetasone
	Topicort gel 0.05%	
	Topicort ointment 0.25%	
III	Aristocort A ointment 0.1%	Triamcinolone acetonide
	Cyclocort cream 0.1%	Amcinonide
	Cyclocort lotion 0.1%	
	Diprosone cream 0.05%	Betamethasone diproprionate
	Florone cream 0.05%	Diflorasone diacetate
	Lidex E Cream 0.05%	Fluocinonide
	Maxiflor cream 0.05%	Diflorasone diacetate
	Maxivate lotion 0.05%	Betamethasone diproprionate
	Valisone ointment 0.1%	Betamethasone valerate

Group	Brand Name	Generic Name
IV	Aristocort ointment 0.1%	Triamcinolone acetonide
	Cordran ointment 0.05%	Flurandrenolide
	Elocon cream 0.1%	Mometasone furoate
	Elocon lotion 0.1%	
	Kenalog cream 0.1%	Triamcinolone acetonide
	Kenalog ointment 0.1%	
	Synalar ointment 0.025%	Fluocinolone acetonide
	Topicort LP cream 0.05%	Desoximelasone
V	Cordran cream 0.05%	Flurandrenolide
	Kenalog lotion 0.1%	Triamcinolone acetonide
	Kenalog ointment 0.025%	
	Locoid cream 0.1%	Hydrocortisone butyrate
	Locoid ointment 0.1%	
	Synalar shampoo/cream 0.01%	Fluocinolone acetonide
	Tridesilon ointment 0.05%	Desonide
	Valisone cream 0.1%	Betamethasone valerate
	Valisone lotion 0.1%	
	Westcort cream 0.2%	Hydrocortisone valerate
	Westcort ointment 0.2%	
VI	Aclovate cream 0.05%	Alclometasone diproprionate
	Aclovate ointment 0.05%	
	Aristocort cream 0.1%	Triamcinolone acetonide
	Kenalog cream 0.025%	Triamcinolone acetonide
	Kenalog lotion 0.025%	
	Locoid solution 0.1%	Hydrocortisone butyrate
	Locorten cream 0.03%	Flumethasone pivolate
	Synalar cream 0.01%	Fluocinolone acetonide
	Synalar solution 0.01%	
	Tridesilon cream 0.05%	Desonide
VII	Hytone cream 1.0%, 2.5%	Hydrocortisone
	Hytone lotion 1.0%, 2.5%	
	Hytone ointment 1.0%, 2.5%	Hydrocortisone Acetate and Pramoxine HCl 1%
	Pramosone cream 1.0%, 2.5%	
	Pramosone lotion 1.0%, 2.5%	and others containing dexametha-sone, flumetholone, prednisolone, methylprednisolone, and betamethasone.
	Pramosone ointment 1.0%, and 2.5%	
	Decaspray (aerosol) 0.04%	Dexamethasone
	Decaderm cream 0.1%	
	Desonide cream, ointment and lotion 0.05%	

- **Nonsteroidal Antiinflammatory Agents (NSAIDS)**
  See *Non Opioid Analgesic Chart* in *Appendix*
  Ibuprofen (Motrin, Advil): 600 - 800 mg PO TID
  Naproxen (Naprosyn): 550 mg PO BID
  Indomethacin (Indocin): 25 - 50 mg PO TID
  Ketorolac (Toradol): 30 mg to 60 mg IM; 30 mg IV
- **Cyclooxygenase II inhibitors**
  Celecoxib (Celebrex): 100 mg PO BID - or - 200 mg PO QD
- **Opioids**
  Dosing information for many opioids is provided in the pain management algorithms
  Butorphanol tartrate (Stadol): 2.0 - 3.0 mg intramuscular or intravenous; 1.0 mg/spray metered dose nasal spray
- **Corticosteroids**
  Dexamethasone (Decadron): 4 to 8 mg of dexamethasone orally; follow up dose in 2 hours with the same strength
  As adjunctive therapy, use 4 - 10 mg IM
- **Antiemetics**
  Chlorpromazine (Thorazine)
  Intravenous administration regimen:
  - Dilute 30 mg chlorpromazine in 50 mL of 0.9% saline
  - Infuse at a rate of 10 mg every 20 minutes
  - Concomitantly administer 250 - 500 mL 0.9% saline over one hour in otherwise healthy adults
  - The patient can become pain-free or asleep after 1 to 3 of the 10 mg doses

  Intramuscular administration: 1 mg/kg IM

  Prochlorperazine (Compazine)
  - Intravenous administration: 10 mg by slow IV injection over 1 to 2 minutes
  - Intramuscular administration: 1 mg/kg IM
  - Rectal administration: 25 mg PR for adults

  Metoclopramide (Reglan): 10 mg or 0.1 mg/kg IV

- **Serotonin Antagonists**

  Ergotamine tartrate: 2 mg PO, followed one hour later by 1 to 2 mg PO. The total daily dose should not exceed 4 mg.

  Dihydroergotamine

  Method I

  - Pre-treat patient with: 10 mg IV or IM prochlorperazine (Compazine) over 2 min or 25 - 50 mg IM promethazine (Phenergan) or 8 to 10 mg chlorpromazine (Thorazine) in 100 mL of 0.9% saline over 30 minutes (good when sleep is desired).
  - 5 to 10 minutes later, administer 0.75 - 1.0 mg IV DHE (2 minute intravenous infusion)
  - If there is no relief from the headache after 1 hour, then administer DHE 0.75 mg intravenous (second dose)*.
  - If no relief after second dose, administer sleep inducing agent such as IV chlorpromazine or an opioid.

  Method II

  - 1 mL (1.0 mg) DHE and 2 mL (10 mg) prochlorperazine (Compazine) in single 3-mL syringe
  - Administer intravenously over 2 minutes.
  - If there is no relief from the headache after 1 hour, then administer DHE 0.75 mg intravenous (second dose).
  - If no relief after second dose, administer sleep inducing agent such as IV chlorpromazine or an opioid.

  * DHE nasal spray (Migranal) is an alternative to IV medication.

- **Other agents:**

  Sumatriptan (Imitrex): 6 mg subcutaneous injection. If still in pain after one hour, repeat 6 mg subcutaneous injection. Imitrex nasal spray (20 mg) and oral tablets are alternatives.

  Naratriptan (Amerge): 1 mg and 2.5 mg tablets

  Zolmitriptan (Zomig): 2.5 - 5.0 mg PO

  Rizatriptan (Maxalt): Refer to manufacturer for dosing information.

  Lidocaine: 0.4 cc of 4% intranasal lidocaine

  Capsaicin: Topical application to nasal mucosa

Suppository recipes

DA Suppository (**D**ecadron **A**tivan)
- Place suppository mold in freezer
- Melt 1/2 cup fattibase or 13 (blank) suppositories
- Crush: Thirty-five (35) 4 mg Decadron (dexamethasone) and fourteen (14) 2 mg Ativan (lorazepam)
- Add drugs and mix well: Makes 14 suppositories
- 3 month expiration
- Each suppository contains 10 mg Decadron (dexamethasone) and 2 mg Ativan (lorazepam)

RDA Suppository (**R**eglan **D**ecadron **A**tivan)
- Melt 1/2 cup fattibase or 13 (blank) suppositories
- Crush: Seventy (70) 10 mg Reglan (metoclopramide), thirty-five (35) 4 mg Decadron (dexamethasone), fourteen (14) 2 mg Ativan (lorazepam)
- Add drugs and mix well: makes 14 suppositories
- 3 months expiration
- Each suppository contains: Reglan (metoclopramide) 50 mg, Decadron (dexamethasone) 10 mg, Ativan (lorazepam) 2 mg

DBR Suppository (**D**ecadron **B**enadryl **R**eglan)
- Place suppository mold in freezer
- Melt 1/2 cup fattibase or 13 (blank) suppositories
- Crush: Thirty-five (35) 4 mg Decadron (dexamethasone), seven (7) 50 mg Benadryl (diphenhydramine), twenty-eight (28) 10 mg Reglan (metoclopramide)
- Add drugs and mix well: makes 14 suppositories
- 3 month expiration
- Each suppository contains 10 mg Decadron (dexamethasone), 25 mg Benadryl (diphenhydramine), 20 mg Reglan (metoclopramide)

Therapy for H. Pylori

A variety of regimens are available to treat gastrointestinal symptoms due to H. Pylori. Selected regimens are listed here. The cost to the pharmacist is based upon the average wholesale price. Other H2 receptor antagonists could be used instead of ranitidine (Zantac). Helidac therapy is supplied as 14 blister cards, each containing eight 262.4 mg bismuth subsalicylate tablets, four 250 mg metronidazole tablets and four 500 mg tetracycline tablets. Tritec is equivalent to 162 mg of ranitidine, 128 mg of trivalent bismuth and 110 mg of citrate. *Medical letter, Vol. 39 (991) January 3, 1997*

Selected Drugs Regimens for treating H. Pylori			
Drugs	Daily Dose	Duration	Cost
Bismuth subsalicylate (generic)	2 tabs (525 mg) QID	2 weeks	10.38
+ Metronidazole (generic)	250 mg QID	2 weeks	1.85
+ Tetracycline (generic)	500 mg QID	2 weeks	3.49
+ Ranitidine (Zantac)	150 mg BID	2 weeks	44.64
			60.36
Helidac Therapy			77.70
+ Ranitidine (Zantac)	150 mg BID	2 weeks	44.64
			122.34
Clarithromycin (Biaxin)	500 mg PID	2 weeks	136.91
+ Omeprazole (Prilosec)	40 mg once	2 weeks	101.64
followed by Omeprazole	20 mg once	2 weeks	50.82
			289.37
Clarithromycin	500 mg BID	10 days	65.20
+ Omeprazole	20 mg BID	10 days	72.60
or Lansoprazole (Prevacid)	15 mg BID	10 days	67.17
+ Metronidazole	500 mg BID	10 days	1.37
or Amoxicillin (generic)	1 gram BID	10 days	9.18
			133.00 -147.00
Ranitidine bismuth citrate (Tritec)	400 mg BID	2 weeks	48.72
+ Clarithromycin	500 mg TID	2 weeks	136.91
followed by ranitidine bismuth citrate	400 mg BID	2 weeks	48.72
			234.35

World Health Organization Analgesic Ladder

Third Step
Always ATC
(Strong Opioids)

Patients who fail step 2 or who present with very severe pain, assess need for adjuvant medications and non-opioid analgesics

Second Step
Always ATC
(Weak Opioids)

Patients who fail step 1 or present with moderate to severe pain, assess need for adjuvant medications and non-opioid analgesics

First Step
May be PRN or ATC
(Non-Opioids)

Patients who present with mild to moderate pain, assess need for adjuvant medications

See associated algorithms for each step.
See adjuvant medication chart.

ATC = around the clock

Pain Assessment Tool

	Scale	
No Pain	0	
	1	
Mild Pain, Annoying	2	
	3	
Nagging Uncomfortable, Troublesome	4	
	5	
Distressing, Miserable	6	
	7	
Intense, Dreadful, Horrible	8	
	9	
Worst Pain Possible, Unbearable, Excruciating	10	

Pain Assessment Form

Frequency of pain interfering with patient's activity or movement:

Score

- [ ] 0 - No problem identified
- [ ] 0 - Patient has no pain or pain does not interfere with activity or movement
- [ ] 1 - Less often than daily
- [ ] 2 - Daily, but not constantly
- [ ] 3 - All the time

Pain intensity as stated by patient

0   1   2   3   4   5   6   7   8   9   10

Indicate patient's personal goal for pain relief

0   1   2   3   4   5   6   7   8   9   10

Location of pain

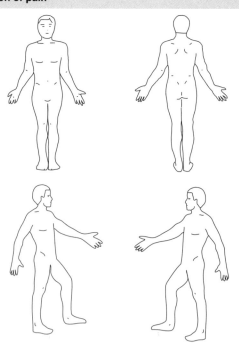

Onset of pain

- [ ] Chronic (2 months or more)
- [ ] Acute (less than one month)

Precipitating factors	Alleviating factors
- [ ] Position changes	- [ ] Lying still
- [ ] Walking	- [ ] Heat
- [ ] Standing	- [ ] Changing positions
- [ ] Temperature changes	- [ ] Cold
- [ ] Range of motion	- [ ] Massage
- [ ] Sitting	- [ ] Medications
- [ ] Breathing	- [ ] Relaxation
- [ ] Other	- [ ] Other

Quality of pain

- [ ] Dull	- [ ] Aching
- [ ] Pressure like	- [ ] Crushing
- [ ] Gnawing	- [ ] Annoying
- [ ] Tight	- [ ] Heavy
- [ ] Tender	- [ ] Throbbing
- [ ] Cramping	- [ ] Nagging
- [ ] Squeezing	- [ ] Uncomfortable
- [ ] Itching	- [ ] Pinching
- [ ] Sharp	- [ ] Pins and needles
- [ ] Shooting	- [ ] Stabbing
- [ ] Lancinating	- [ ] Burning
- [ ] Stinging	- [ ] Tingling
	- [ ] Other

Cause of Pain   Comments

- [ ] Known   _____
- [ ] Unknown   _____

What does the patient feel is causing the pain?

_____
_____

Associated symptoms

☐ Constipation	☐ Sedation
☐ Confusion	☐ Depression
☐ Irritability	☐ Sleep disruption
☐ Anorexia	☐ Nausea
☐ Anxiety	☐ Agitation
☐ Spiritual distress	☐ Feelings of hopelessness
☐ Suicidal ideation	☐ Fear
☐ Isolation/loneliness	☐ Guilt
	☐ Other

Intractable pain: Is the patient experiencing pain that is not easily relieved, occurs at least daily, and affects the patient's sleep, appetite, physical or emotional energy, concentration, personal relationships, emotions, or ability/desire to perform physical activity?

☐ No
☐ Yes

Meaning of pain: What would you do if you did not have pain? How are your activities of daily living impacted by your pain? How is your relationship with others impacted by pain? How do others perceive your pain? What expectations do you have regarding pain relief? What are realistic goals for you?

_____
_____
_____
_____

Location of pain

_____
_____
_____
_____

_____

Patient Name

Pain Management Principles

- Believe the patient's report of pain
- By the mouth (whenever possible)
- By the clock (around the clock rather than PRN)
- By the ladder (WHO analgesic ladder)
- Provide rescue doses
- Use adjuvant medications
- Titrate to effect
- Use equianalgesic doses
- Don't forget the non-pharmacologic modalities: heat relaxation, cold, imagery, massage, TENS, music, biofeedback, humor, acupressure, acupuncture, aromatherapy, therapeutic touch
- Treat side effects vigorously
- Use multidisciplinary approach
- Keep it simple
- Progress in a systematic fashion
    - Oral (preferred route)
    - Transdermal
    - Sublingual/Transmucosal
    - Rectal/Vaginal/Ostomy
    - PCA (Patient controlled analgesia)
        - Subcutaneous (preferred route)
        - IV (only if there is a vascular access device already in place)
        - Epidural (useful in about 10%)
        - Intrathecal
        - Intracerebral ventricular ports
- Modify pathologic process when feasible
- Consult specialist when indicated
- Immobilize when necessary
- Interrupt pain pathways
- Avoid fixed dose combinations; they are hard to titrate
- Most opioids have no known ceiling except meperidine (Demerol) and methadone (Dolophine); these agents have limitations due to the accumulation of active metabolites
- Most drugs achieve a steady state after five doses
- Try and keep on trying

Pain Descriptions

Key elements of pain assessment:
- Location
- Quality
- Intensity (use 1-10 scale)
- Onset
- Duration
- Alleviating factors
- Aggravating factors
- History of present illness
- Frequency (constant, intermittent, transient)
- Radiation
- Meaning of pain
  (impact on patient's function and quality of life)
- What co-morbid conditions exist

PQRST mnemonic: **P**=palliative or precipitating factors; **Q** = Quality of Life impact; **R**=Radiation/distribution of pain; **S**=Severity of pain; **T**=Temporal patterning; **U**=You: impact on the patient's life.
(PQRST mnemonic per American Pharmaceutical Association)

Suggested questions:

What is the quality of your pain?

What word or words describe your pain?

- See Pain Assessment Form in Appendix
- See Quality of Life Scoring tools in the Appendix

Specific pain descriptions

Dull, aching, pressure-like, crushing, gnawing, boring, tight, heavy, tender, throbbing, squeezing, cutting, tingling, flickering, itching, stinging, pinching, cramping, sharp, shooting stabbing, lancinating, burning, continuous, steady, constant, rhythmic, periodic, intermittent, brief, momentary, transient

---

Impact on Quality of Life Parameters
- Overall activity
- Mood
- Ability to walk
- Ability to work
- Ability to eat or drink
- Relationships with people
- Sleep
- Enjoyment of life

Pain Syndromes

1. Nociceptive: actual or potential tissue damage.

    a. Somatic: skin, muscle, bone -- aching, stabbing, throbbing, pressure-like

    b. Visceral: internal organs -- gnawing or cramping when due to obstruction of hollow viscus; aching, sharp, or throbbing when due to involvement of organ capsules

    c. Nerve damage: aching, sharp, throbbing

2. Neuropathic: aberrant sensations in the peripheral or central nervous system (dysesthesia, abnormal unfamiliar pain, burning, shooting, "pins and needles")

3. Affective/idiopathic: perceived to be excessive in relation to the disease process present. Psychological and behavioral disturbances such as anxiety and agitation may coexist.

4. Iatrogenic: pain induced by therapeutic maneuvers

5. Other syndromes

    • Chronic pain syndrome (greater than six months)

    • Musculoskeletal pain syndrome

    • Headache syndromes

Diagnosis of type of pain is important since nociceptive (somatic/visceral) pain responds well to opioids and NSAIDS whereas neuropathic pain often does not.

Pain management options

Pain management options when opioid therapy is limited by intolerable dose related side effects:

• Use of adjuvants often decreases systemic opioid use.

• Aggressive management of side effects (See *Opioid Induced Sedation Algorithm*).

• Epidural opioids (often a tenth of IV dosage requirement).

• Appropriate use of more aggressive procedures such as neuroablation, cryoanalgesia, radiofrequency, cordotomy, intracerebral stimulation or surgery.

• Conversion to a different opioid, noting possible cross tolerance.

• Optimize non pharmacologic approaches, use of physio-therapy and rehabilitation services, psychological adjuncts such as hypnosis or distraction therapy and spiritual supports.

Pearls For Analgesic Titration

Analgesic Titration: Pearls of Successful Management

- The doses listed in the Equianalgesic Chart should not be interpreted as the starting, standard or maximum dose. Use as a guide when switching drugs or changing routes of administration. Titrating doses upward or downward is the norm.

- Patient characteristics (disease state, differences in absorption, organ dysfunction and prior opioid exposure/tolerance) will impact the starting dose of a particular analgesic.

- Knowledge of the onset, peak effect and duration of action and half-life of each analgesic will enhance one's ability to skillfully and safely titrate analgesics to achieve optimal analgesia with minimal side effects.

- Be aware of potential drug interactions.

- The intramuscular route for around the clock dosing is *not* recommended; it is painful and absorption is inconsistent.

- The oral route is the preferred route as long as there is an intact, functioning GI tract. The subcutaneous route is the recommended alternate route, especially for quick titration. Transdermal, transmucosal, or intravenous (if IV line is already in place) are good alternatives.

- The keys to safe titration of opioids, regardless of the route of administration are as follows:

    - Thorough and frequent pain assessments
    - Careful monitoring of the patient's response to the drug
    - Start low and go slow especially in the frail or elderly.

- Titrate by percents rather than by milligrams.

- When titrating an intravenous or subcutaneous dose don't forget to add in breakthrough dosages. Example: The basal rate is morphine 5 mg/hr; the PCA dose is 2.5 mg every 10 minutes PRN. After 1 hour the patient has received 5 PCA doses. The respiratory rate is 22. The pain score is 8/10; the patient is alert, oriented and talking coherently. Add up the total milligrams the patient received in the past hour: 5 mg + (5 x 2.5 mg) =17.5 mg. Adjust the new basal rate to 17.5 mg/hr plus 9 mg (9 mg is approximately 50% of the hourly rate) every 10 minutes PRN. Reassess patient for sedation and pain score every hour until pain is less than or equal to 5/10 then every 2-3 hours until pain is less than or equal to 3/10. Remember, sedation precedes respiratory depression.

Pearls For Analgesic Titration

- If the pain score is less than 5/10 with no sedation, titrate upward by 25-50%. For scores over 5/10, titrate up by 50-100%.

- If the pain score is less than 5/10 and there is sedation, titrate downward by 25%. For scores over 5/10, titrate up by 25% with caution.

- Rarely, a naloxone (Narcan) drip may be needed to balance pain control and sedation. Other options include switching to another opioid, adding an adjuvant drug so that opioid dose can be reduced, or adding a stimulant (See *Opioid Induced Sedation* and *Adjuvant Medication Guide* in the *Appendix*)

- To titrate oral opioids, use an immediate release formulation of any formulation such as morphine (MSIR). Give the dose every 1 - 2 hours until pain is less than 3/10. Then convert to a long acting opioid such as MS Contin and Oxycontin. Add a fast acting opioid for breakthrough pain (BTP). Continue to titrate based on the total 24-hour requirement to maintain pain score at less than 3/10 with minimal side effects.

- MS Contin and Oxycontin can be titrated safely every 24 hours. The breakthrough pain dose is calculated to be 25 - 33% of the Q 12 h dose. Titrate upward until the patient is comfortable, pain scores are less than 3/10 or the patient is using less than 3 break though pain doses in a 24 hour period.

- Transdermal fentanyl patches (Duragesic) are a good option once the pain is stabilized with an oral or parenteral opioid. Patients with poorly controlled pain should be treated with a fast acting opioid (such as transmucosal/intravenous fentanyl, oral morphine sulfate, or oxycodone) prior to switching to a transdermal system. Titrate patches after initial 72 hours, then every cycle (3-6 days) depending on use of breakthrough medications.

- Note: Transdermal fentanyl patches are not intended for acute post operative pain, nor for patients who need only intermittent PRN opioids to maintain pain control. Patches are contraindicated in patients weighing less than 110 pounds (50 kg). Use cautiously with the frail or elderly.

Equianalgesic Conversion Guide

Drug	Onset (mins)	Peak (hours)	Duration (hours)	Half-life (hours)
Morphine	15 to 30	0.5 to 1	3 to 7	2 to 4
Levorphanol	30 to 90	0.5 to 1	4 to 8	12 to 16
Hydromorphone	15 to 30	0.5 to 1	4 to 5	2 to 3
Oxymorphone	5 to 10	0.5 to 1	3 to 6	2 to 4
Methadone	30 to 60	0.5 to 1	4 to 8	15 to 120
Meperidine	10 to 45	0.5 to 1	2 to 4	3 to 4
Fentanyl IM	7 to 8	-	1 to 2	1.5 to 6
Fentanyl TM	5 to 15	0.3 to 0.5	5 to 15	2 to 4
Fentanyl IV	Immediate	< 1 min	1 to 2	1 to 4
Fentanyl TD	Slow	18-24	48-72	variable*
Codeine	15 to 30	0.5 to 1	4 to 6	3
Oxycodone	15 to 30	0.5 to 1	2 to 5	3 to 4
Propoxyphene (PO)	30 to 60	2 to 2.5	4 to 6	6 to 12
Hydrocodone	10 to 20	0.5 to 1	4 to 8	3.3 to 4.5
Buprenorphine	10 to 30	0.5 to 1	6 to 8	2 to 3
Tramadol	15 to 30	0.5 to 1	4 to 6	no data

The equianalgesic conversion guide is not based upon controlled studies; dosages are based upon single dose studies in opioid naive patients with acute pain, starting with low dose opioids.

*Variable half-life of transdermal fentanyl depends upon skin thickness, subcutaneous fat, body temperature, age and hepatorenal function.

Equianalgesic Dosing Guide

	Equianalgesic Doses	
Drug	IM (mg)	Oral (mg)
Morphine	10	30 - 60
Levorphanol	2	4
Hydromorphone	1.5	7.5
Oxymorphone	1	6
Methadone	10	20
Meperidine	75	300
Fentanyl IM	0.1 - 0.4	no data
Codeine	130	200
Oxycodone	15	30
Propoxyphene (PO)	no data	130
Hydrocodone	no data	30
Buprenorphine	0.3	0.8
Tramadol	100	120

The equianalgesic dosing guide is not based upon controlled studies; dosages are based upon single dose studies in opioid naive patients with acute pain, starting with low dose opioids.

Hospice Referral Guidelines for Non-Cancer Diagnoses

- Two or more items marked *yes* should generate a hospice consultation
- Adapted from Am J of Hospice and Palliative Care; Sept/Oct 1997, NHO guidelines

Y	N	General Guidelines
		Life-limiting condition(s), Karnofsky score > 70
		Progression of disease(s)
		Need for frequent hospitalization, office, or ER visits
		Dependence in most ADL's (activities of daily living)
		Weight loss > 10 % over past 6 months
		Serum albumin < 2.5 g/dL
		Cholesterol < 156 mg/d - or - Hct < 41 mg/dL

Y	N	End-Stage Lung Disease - (e.g. COPD)
		Dyspnea at rest
		FEV 1 < 30% after bronchodilators
		Recurrent pulmonary infections
		Cor pulmonale/right heart failure
		$pO_2 < 55$ mm Hg - or - O_2 sat < 88% (on O_2)
		Cardiogenic embolic disease (e.g. CVA)
		Persistent resting tachycardia

Y	N	End-Stage Renal Disease
		Creatinine Clearance <10 cc/min (<15 cc/min in diabetics)
		Creatinine > 8 mg/dL (> 6 mg/dL in diabetics)
		Not a candidate for dialysis, renal transplant
		Signs of uremia (confusion, nausea, pruritus, restlessness)
		Oliguria < 400 cc / 24 hrs
		Hyperkalemia > 7.0 mEq / L

Y	N	End-Stage Neurologic Disease (e.g. ALS, Dementia)
		Unable to walk, needs assistance in all ADLs
		Barely intelligible speech
		Nutritional status declining
		Declines feeding tube
		Significant dyspnea on O_2

Y	N	End-Stage Heart Disease (e.g. CHF, CAD)
		Functional Class III & IV NYHA Assessment
		Symptomatic despite maximum medical management with diuretics and vasodilators
		Arrhythmia is resistant to treatment
		Ejection fraction < 20%
		History of cardiac arrest
		Cardiogenic embolic disease (e.g. CVA)
		Persistent resting tachycardia

For patients with non-cancer diagnoses, some may not meet criteria for hospice enrollment, yet still be hospice appropriate because of other comorbidities and rapid decline.

Hospice Referral Guidelines for Non-Cancer Diagnoses

Y	N	**End Stage Liver Disease**
		Not a candidate for liver transplant
		PTT > 5 seconds above control
		Ascites despite maximum diuretics
		Peritonitis
		Hepatorenal syndrome
		Encephalopathy with asterixis, somnolence, coma
		Recurrent variceal bleeding

Y	N	**End-Stage Dementia (AIDS or Multi-infarct)**
		FAST score of 7 (See FAST Score in the Appendix)
		Unable to walk without assistance
		Increasing incontinence
		Speech limited to less than or equal to 6 words per day
		Unable to dress or bathe
		Unable to sit up or hold head up
		Medical complications: recurrent aspiration, pneumonia
		UTI, sepsis, advanced decubiti

Y	N	**CVA and Coma**
		Level of consciousness decreasing
		Persistant vegetative state
		Dysphagia
		Age > 70
		Dependence in activities of daily living, paralysis
		Post stroke dementia
		Nutritional status down (despite feeding tube, if present)
		Medical complications increasing (recurrent, frequent)

Y	N	**AIDS**
		CD4 < 25 / mL
		CD4 > 50 / mL plus non-HIV comorbidities
		Viral load > 100,000 / mL and steady decline
		Viral load < 100,000 / mL plus complications as below
		Wasting Syndrome
		CNS lymphoma
		PML (progressive multifocal leukoencephalopathy)
		Cryptosporidiosis
		MAC (mycobacterium avium complex)
		Visceral Kaposi's sarcoma, unresponsive to treatment
		AIDS dementia
		Toxoplasmosis
		Pneumocystis carinii pneumonia
		Tuberculosis
		Current substance abuse
		Age > 50

Ethical Decision Making Guidelines

Think about the situation objectively
- Clearly understand the situation
- Know the facts
- Identify the real issues

Recognize and analyze motivations
- If the situation troubles you, ask yourself why
- Consider the other party's motivation

Understand your agency's policy and applicable laws.
- Consider all options
- Know whom and when to ask for help if you're unsure

Satisfy the headline test.
- Ask yourself if you'd feel comfortable seeing your actions reported in the news
- Think about how your family and colleagues would feel about your decision
- Consider the consequences of your decision on your patients/ families, on your agency, on your family, on yourself

Take responsibility for your actions
- Make an appropriate choice and act accordingly
- Remember, you are accountable for the outcome of your decisions
- Notify your supervisor when appropriate

Providence Yakima Medical Center Home Care Services
Policy and Procedure Manual on Ethical Guidelines

Staging of pressure ulcers

Staging of pressure ulcers

Stage 1
- Partial thickness wound
- Nonblanchable erythema of intact skin; a heralding lesion of skin ulceration

Stage 2
- Partial thickness skin loss involving epidermis and/or dermis
- The ulcer is superficial and presents clinically as an abrasion, blister, or shallow crater

Stage 3
- Full thickness skin loss involving damage or necrosis of subcutaneous tissue that extends down to, but not through underlying fascia
- The ulcer presents clinically as a deep crater with or without undermining of adjacent tissue

Stage 4
- Full thickness skin loss with extensive destruction, tissue necrosis or damage to muscle, bone, or supporting structures (for example: tendon or joint capsule)
- Undermining of adjacent tissue and sinus tracts may also be present

Unable to stage
- When the wound bed is coverd by 50% or more with necrotic tissue or eschar determining the actual depth is not accurate; therefore it is listed as *unable to stage*

Palliative Performance Scale PPS

%	Ambulation	Activity and Evidence of Disease
100	Full	Normal activity; no evidence of disease
90	Full	Normal activity; some evidence of disease
80	Full	Normal activity with effort; some evidence of disease
70	Reduced	Unable normal job/work; some evidence of disease
60	Reduced	Unable hobby/house work; significant disease
50	Mainly Sit/Lie	Unable to do any work; extensive disease
40	Mainly in Bed	Unable to do any work; extensive disease
30	Totally Bed Bound	Unable to do any work; extensive disease
20	Totally Bed Bound	Unable to do any work; extensive disease
10	Totally Bed Bound	Unable to do any work; extensive disease
0	Death	———

This scale is a modification of the Karnofsky Performance Scale. The PPS takes into account ambulation, activity, self-care, intake and level of consciousness.

www.Intelli-card.com

Palliative Performance Scale PPS

Self-Care	Intake	Conscious Level
Full	Normal	Full
Full	Normal	Full
Full	Normal or reduced	Full
Full	Normal or reduced	Full
Occasional Assistance Necessary	Normal or reduced	Full or Confusion
Considerable Assistance Required	Normal or reduced	Full or Confusion
Mainly Assistance	Normal or reduced	Full or Drowsy or Confusion
Total Care	Reduced	Full or Drowsy or Confusion
Total Care	Minimal Sips	Full or Drowsy or Confusion
Total Care	Mouth Care Only	Drowsy or Coma
—	—	—

ECOG/Karnofsky Functional Rating Scale

ECOG SCALE ECOG = Eastern Cooperative Oncology Group	KARNOFSKY RATING
Grade: 0	100 Able to carry on normal activity; no special care
Grade: 0	90
Grade: 1	80
Grade: 1	70 Unable to work; able to live at home; cares for most personal needs; a varying amount of assistance is needed.
Grade: 2	60
Grade: 2	50
Grade: 3	40 Unable to care for self; requires equivalent of institutional or hospital care; disease may be progressing rapidly.
Grade: 3	30
Grade: 4	20
Grade: 4	10
Grade: 4	1
Grade: 5	0

ECOG/Karnofsky Functional Rating Scale

BEHAVIORS

Normal; no complaints. No evidence of disease. Able to carry on all predisease activities without restriction.

Able to carry on normal activity; minor signs or symptoms of disease.

Normal activity with effort Some signs or symptoms of disease. Restricted in strenuous physical activity but ambulatory and able to carry out work of a sedentary nature, e.g. light housework, office work.

Cares for self. Unable to carry out normal home chores or to do active work.

Requires occasional assistance but is able to care for most of self care needs. Ambulatory and capable of all self care but unable to carry out any work activities. Up and about more than 50% of waking hours.

Requires considerable assistance and frequent medical care.

Disabled; requires special care and assistance. Capable of only limited self-care; confined to bed or chair more than 50% of waking hours.

Severely disabled; although death is not imminent, hospital-like care is indicated.

Very sick; hospital like care necessary. Completely disabled. Cannot carry on any self-care. Totally confined to bed or chair.

Moribund; fatal processes progressing rapidly.

Unconscious

Dead

NYHA Functional Classification

NEW YORK HEART ASSOCIATION (NYHA) FUNCTIONAL CLASSIFICATION	
CLASS I	Patients with cardiac disease; no limitations of physical activity
	Ordinary physical activity does not cause undue fatigue, palpitations, dyspnea, or anginal pain
CLASS II	Patients with cardiac disease and only slight limitation of physical activity; comfortable at rest
	Ordinary physical activity results in fatigue, palpitations, dyspnea, or anginal pain
CLASS III	Patients with cardiac disease with marked limitation of physical activity; comfortable at rest
	Less than ordinary activity causes fatigue, palpitations, dyspnea, or anginal pain
CLASS IV	Patients with cardiac disease resulting in inability to carry on any physical activity without discomfort
	Symptoms of heart failure or anginal syndrome at rest. If any physical activity is undertaken, discomfort is increased

For any patient enrolled in hospice with an automatic implantable defibrillator, the plan of care should address the issue of continuation, deactivation or adjustment in consultation with the patient's cardiologist in accordance with the patient's directive.

FAST Score

Functional Assessment Staging (FAST)

- **Check Highest Consecutive Level of Disability**
- **Hospice Appropriate if FAST score 6 or 7**

1	No difficulty either subjectively or objectively
2	Complains of forgetting location of objects Subjective work difficulties*
3	Decreased job functioning evident to co-workers Difficulty in traveling to new locations. Decreased organization capacity*
4	Decreased ability to perform complex tasks such as:* • Planning dinner for guests • Handling personal finances (e.g. forgetting to pay bills) • Difficulty shopping, etc.
5	Requires assistance in choosing proper clothing to wear for the day, season or occasion* Repeatedly, observed wearing the same clothing, unless supervised
6	Improperly putting on clothes without assistance or cueing* (e.g. may put street clothes on overnight clothes, put shoes on wrong feet, have difficulty buttoning clothing) Unable to bathe properly (e.g. difficulty adjusting bath-water temperature)* Unable to handle mechanics of toileting (e.g. forgets to flush the toilet, does not wipe properly or properly dispose of toilet tissue)* Urinary incontinence* Fecal incontinence*
7	Limited ability to speak ≤ 6 intelligible different words in an average day or interview* Speech ability is limited to the use of a single intelligible word in a normal interaction. Repetitive actions.* Ambulatory ability is lost (cannot walk without personal assistance) Cannot sit up without assistance* Individual falls over if no lateral arm rests on chair* Loss of ability to smile* Loss of ability to hold up head independently*

*Occasionally or more frequently over the past weeks

Mini-Mental Status Examination

Instructions for Administration

Make the patient comfortable, establish rapport, and praise success.

Ask questions in the order listed and score immediately.

Total possible score is 30.

ORIENTATION

(1) Time orientation (Ask *Year, Season, Date, Day, Month*)

(2) Orientation to place (Ask *State, County, Town*)

REGISTRATION

Ask the patient if you may test his/her memory. Then say the names of 3 unrelated objects, clearly and slowly, about one second for each. (For example: *ball, pencil, comb*) After you have said all 3, ask him/her to repeat them. The first repetition determines the score (3-3), but keep saying them until he/she can repeat all 3, up to 5 trials. Otherwise, recall cannot be meaningfully tested.

ATTENTION AND CALCULATION

Ask the patient to begin with 100 and count backwards by 7. Stop after 5 subtractions (93, 86, 79, 72, 65). Score the total number of correct answers.

If the patient cannot or will not perform the Serial 7's task, ask him/her to spell the word "*WORLD*" backwards. Score the number of letters in correct order. e.g. DLROW - 5, DLORW = 3.

RECALL

Ask the patient if he/she can recall the 3 words previously asked to remember. Score 0-3.

LANGUAGE

Naming: Show the patient a wristwatch and ask him/her what it is. Repeat for pencil. Score 0-2.

Repetition: Ask the patient to repeat the phrase after you. Allow only one trial. Score 0 or 1.

3-Stage Command: Give the patient a piece of blank paper and repeat the command. Score 1 point for each part correctly executed.

Reading: On a blank piece of paper, print the sentence *CLOSE YOUR EYES* in letters large enough for the patient to see clearly. Ask him/her to read it and do what it says.

Writing: Give the patient a blank piece of paper and ask him/her to write a sentence for you. Do not dictate a sentence; it is to be written spontaneously. It must contain a subject and verb and be sensible. Correct grammar and punctuation are not necessary.

Copying: Ask the patient to copy the figure of the intersecting pentagons exactly as it is. All 10 angles must be present and 2 must intersect to form a 4-sided figure to score 1 point. Tremor and rotation are ignored.

Mini-Mental Status Examination

Maximum score	Score	
		ORIENTATION
5	( )	What is the (*Year*) (*Season*) (*Date*) (*Day*) (*Month*)? *One point for each correct response*
5	( )	Where are we: (*State*) (*County*) (*Town* or *City*) (*Hospital*) (*Floor*)? *One point for each correct response*
		REGISTRATION
3	( )	NAME 3 COMMON OBJECTS (eg, *apple, table, penny*) *One point for each correct response* Count trials and record. Trials:
		ATTENTION AND CALCULATION
5	( )	Serial 7"s , backwards. *One point for each correct response* Stop after 5 answers. Alternatively, spell "WORLD" backwards. *One point for each correct response*
		RECALL
3	( )	Ask for the 3 objects repeated above. *One point for each correct response*
		LANGUAGE
2	( )	Name a pencil and a watch.
1	( )	Repeat the following: *"No ifs, ands, or buts."*
3	( )	Follow a 3 stage command: *Take a paper in your right hand, fold it in half, and put it on the floor.* *One point for each part correctly executed.*
1	( )	Read and obey the following: **CLOSE YOUR EYES**
1	( )	Write a sentence.
1	( )	Copy the following design

Severity of cognitive impairments
Mild: MMSE ≥ 21 **Moderate:** MMSE 10-20 **Severe**: MMSE ≤ 9
The expected decline in MMSE scores in untreated mild to moderate
Alzheimer's patients is 2 to 4 points per year.

Quality of Life Assessment Guidelines

Critcal features of a quality of life assesment tool

- A well-defined global construct that has clinical applicability.
- Self-reported rather than observer-rated; a subjective assessment.
- A multidimensional construct that assesses relevant spheres of personhood, especially those related to health, function, and the psychological, emotional and spiritual dimensions of self.
- Ability to weight personal dimensions and create a scoring methodology.
- Ability to measure changes experienced by the person in both negative and positive directions from pre-illness status (i.e. create a baseline within each dimension) preferably on a day to day basis.
- Reportable scores (total and dimensional components) that are clinically meaningful.
- Sensibility which includes measurements of reliability, validity as well as "real world" applicability and utility.*
- Ease of administration, scoring, and interpretation.
- Use as a discriminative tool, measuring differences between groups of persons.
- Use as an evaluative tool, designed for repeated use, measuring changes in an individual over a period of time.
- Tool to be adopted in a culturally sensitive format.

Feinstein AR. Clinimetrics. New Haven, CT: Yale University Press, 1987: 141-66

*Adapted from Melanie P Merriman, VITAS Healthcare Corporation, 100 S. Biscayne Blvd., Suite 1500, Miami, FL 33131, USA Palliative Medicine 1998; 12: 231-244

Quality of Life Assessment Guidelines-MVQOL

MVQOL = Missoula-VITAS ® quality of life index version -25S

Quality of Life dimensions screened by the MVQOLI

SYMPTOM (S):	The level of physical discomfort and distress experienced with progressive illness.
FUNCTION (F):	Perceived ability to perform accustomed functions and activities of daily living and the emotional response, experienced in relation to the person's expectations.
INTERPERSONAL (IP):	Degree of investment in personal relationships and the perceived quality of ones relations/interactions with family and friends.
WELL-BEING (WB): (Intrapersonal)	Self-assessment of the individual's internal condition. A subjective sense of wellness, unease, contentment or lack of contentment
TRANSCENDENT (T): (Transpersonal)	The degree of connection one has with an enduring construct; the meaning and purpose to one's life

Self Reported Assessments of the QOL dimensions

SELF ASSESSMENT (A):	Subjective measurement of one's actual status or circumstance. Example: I feel sick all the time.
SATISFACTION (S):	Feelings or emotions in response to actual circumstances. Example: I accept my symptoms as a fact of life.
IMPORTANCE (I):	The degree to which a given dimension has an impact on quality of life. Example: Despite my physical discomfort, I can enjoy my days.

Palliative Medicine 1998; 12: 231-244

Missoula - VITAS ® quality of life index version - 25S

Instructions

Indicate the extent to which you agree or disagree with the following statements by filling in ONE of the circles along the line. For items with two statements choose a circle close to the statement with which you agree more. If you make a mistake or change your mind, mark an X through the wrong answer, and fill in the circle indicating your correct answer. Please fill in the circle completely.

Global

How would you rate your overall quality of life?

Best Possible ←   O O O O O   → Worst Possible

Symptom

1. My symptoms are adequately controlled.

   Agree ←   O O O O O   → Disagree

2. I feel sick all the time.

   Agree ←   O O O O O   → Disagree

3. I accept my symptoms as a fact of life.

   Agree ←   O O O O O   → Disagree

4. I am satisfied with the current control of my symptoms.

   Agree ←   O O O O O   → Disagree

5. Despite physical discomfort , in general I can enjoy my days

   Physical discomfort overshadows any opportunity for enjoyment

   Agree ←   O O O O O   → Agree

Function

6. I am still able to attend most of my personal needs by myself.

   I am dependent on others for personal care.

   Agree ←   O O O O O   → Agree

7. I am still able to do
many of the things I
like to do.

   I am no longer able
to do many of the
things I like to do.

   Agree ← ○ ○ ○ ○ ○ → Agree

8. I am satisfied with my ability to take care of my basic needs.

   Agree ← ○ ○ ○ ○ ○ → Disagree

9. I accept the fact
that I can not do
many things that I
used to do.

   I am disappointed that I
can not do many of the
things that I used to do.

   Agree ← ○ ○ ○ ○ ○ → Agree

10. My contentment with life depends upon being active and being
independent in my personal care.

   Agree ← ○ ○ ○ ○ ○ → Disagree

Interpersonal

11. I have recently been able to say important things to the people
close to me.

   Agree ← ○ ○ ○ ○ ○ → Disagree

12. I feel closer to others in
my life now than I did
before my illness.

   I feel increasingly
distant from others in
my life.

   Agree ← ○ ○ ○ ○ ○ → Agree

13. In general, these days I am satisfied with relationships with
family and friends.

   Agree ← ○ ○ ○ ○ ○ → Disagree

14. At present, I spend as much time as I want with family and
friends.

   Agree ← ○ ○ ○ ○ ○ → Disagree

15. It is important to me to have close personal relationships.

   Agree ← ○ ○ ○ ○ ○ → Disagree

Well-being

16. My affairs are in order; I could die today with a clear mind.

    My affairs are not in order; I am worried that many things are unresolved.

    Agree ← ○ ○ ○ ○ ○ → Agree

17. I feel generally at peace and prepared to leave this life.

    I am unsettled and unprepared to leave this life.

    Agree ← ○ ○ ○ ○ ○ → Agree

18. I am more satisfied with myself as a person now than I was before my illness.

    Agree ← ○ ○ ○ ○ ○ → Disagree

19. The longer I am ill, the more I worry about things getting out of control

    The longer I am ill, the more comfortable I am with the idea of letting go

    Agree ← ○ ○ ○ ○ ○ → Agree

20. It is important to me to be at peace with myself.

    Agree ← ○ ○ ○ ○ ○ → Disagree

Transcendent

21. I have a greater sense of connection to all things now than I did before my illness.

    I feel more disconnected from all things now than I did before my illness.

    Agree ← ○ ○ ○ ○ ○ → Agree

22. I have a better sense of meaning in my life now than I have had in the past.

I have less of a sense of meaning in my life now than I have had in the past.

Agree ← ○ ○ ○ ○ ○ → Agree

23. As the end of my life approaches, I am comfortable with the thought of my own death.

As the end of my life approaches, I am uneasy with the thought of my own death.

Agree ← ○ ○ ○ ○ ○ → Agree

24. Life has become more precious to me; every day is a gift.

Life has lost all value for me; every day is a burden.

Agree ← ○ ○ ○ ○ ○ → Agree

25. It is important to me to feel that my life has meaning.

Agree ← ○ ○ ○ ○ ○ → Disagree

Did you complete this questionaire by yourself?

○ Yes   No ○

Quality of Life Linear Analog Score

Quality of Life - Linear analog scale assessment
(to be completed by the patient)

There are three questions about how the patient felt during this past week. Have the patient place a vertical mark on the line to indicate the answer. The position of the mark, somewhere between the two extremes, should reflect how the patient feels.

1. How would you rate your energy level during the past week?

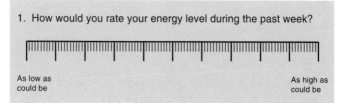

As low as
could be   As high as
                                           could be

2. How would you rate your ability to do your daily activities over the past week?

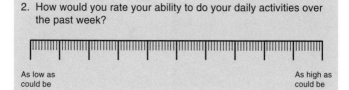

As low as
could be   As high as
                                           could be

3. How would you rate your overall quality of life during the past week?

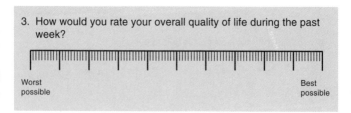

Worst
possible   Best
                                           possible

FACT Score

Below is a list of statements that other people with your illness have said are important. By circling one number per line, please indicate how true each statement has been for you during the past 7 days.

	Not at all	A little bit	Somewhat	Quite a bit	Very much

Physical well being

		Not at all	A little bit	Somewhat	Quite a bit	Very much
1.	I have a lack of energy	0	1	2	3	4
2.	I have nausea	0	1	2	3	4
3.	Because of my physical condition, I have trouble meeting the needs of my family	0	1	2	3	4
4.	I have pain	0	1	2	3	4
5.	I am bothered by side effects of treatment	0	1	2	3	4
6.	I feel sick	0	1	2	3	4
7.	I am forced to spend time in bed	0	1	2	3	4
8.	Looking at the above 7 questions, how much would you say your physical well-being affects your quality of life?	1 2 3 4 5 6 7 8 9 10				

Social / Family Well Being

		Not at all	A little bit	Somewhat	Quite a bit	Very much
9.	I feel distant from my friends	0	1	2	3	4
10.	I get emotional support from my family	0	1	2	3	4
11.	I get support from my friends and neighbors	0	1	2	3	4
12.	My family has accepted my illness	0	1	2	3	4
13.	Family communication about my illness is poor	0	1	2	3	4
14.	I feel close to my partner (or the person who is my main support)	0	1	2	3	4
15.	Have you been sexually active during the past year? Y/N If yes, I am satisfied with my sex life.	0	1	2	3	4
16.	Looking at the above 7 questions, how much would you say your social/family well-being affects your quality of life? (circle one)	1 2 3 4 5 6 7 8 9 10				

FACT Score

	Not at all	A little bit	Somewhat	Quite a bit	Very much

Relationship with doctor

		Not at all	A little bit	Somewhat	Quite a bit	Very much
17.	I have confidence in my doctor(s)	0	1	2	3	4
18.	My doctor is available to answer my questions	0	1	2	3	4
19.	Looking at the above 2 questions, how much would you say your relationship with the doctor affect your well-being	1 2 3 4 5 6 7 8 9 10				

Emotional well-being

		Not at all	A little bit	Somewhat	Quite a bit	Very much
20.	I feel sad	0	1	2	3	4
21.	I am proud of how I'm coping with my illness	0	1	2	3	4
22.	I am losing hope in the fight against my illness	0	1	2	3	4
23.	I feel nervous	0	1	2	3	4
24.	I worry about dying	0	1	2	3	4
25.	I worry that my condition will get worse	0	1	2	3	4
26.	Looking at the above 6 questions, how much would you say your emotional well-being affects your quality of life?	1 2 3 4 5 6 7 8 9 10				

Functional Well-being

		Not at all	A little bit	Somewhat	Quite a bit	Very much
27.	I am able to work (include work in home)	0	1	2	3	4
28.	My work (include work in home) is fulfilling	0	1	2	3	4
29.	I am able to enjoy life	0	1	2	3	4
30.	I have accepted my illness	0	1	2	3	4
31.	I am sleeping well					
32.	I am enjoying the things I usually do for fun	0	1	2	3	4
33.	I am content with the quality of my life right now	0	1	2	3	4
34.	Looking at the above 7 questions, how much would you say your functional well-being affects your quality of life? (circle one)	1 2 3 4 5 6 7 8 9 10				

FACT Score

	Not at all	A little bit	Somewhat	Quite a bit	Very much
Additional concerns					
35. I feel fatigued	0	1	2	3	4
36. I feel weak all over	0	1	2	3	4
37. I feel listless ("washed out")	0	1	2	3	4
38. I feel tired	0	1	2	3	4
39. I have trouble starting things because I am tired	0	1	2	3	4
40. I have trouble finishing things because I am tired	0	1	2	3	4
41. I have energy	0	1	2	3	4
42. I have trouble walking	0	1	2	3	4
43. I am able to do my usual activities	0	1	2	3	4
44. I need to sleep during the day	0	1	2	3	4
45. I feel light-headed (dizzy)	0	1	2	3	4
46. I get headaches	0	1	2	3	4
47. I have been short of breath	0	1	2	3	4
48. I have pain in my chest	0	1	2	3	4
49. I am too tired to eat	0	1	2	3	4
50. I am interested in sex	0	1	2	3	4
51. I am motivated to do my usual activities	0	1	2	3	4
52. I need help doing my usual activities	0	1	2	3	4
53. I am frustrated by being too tired to do the things I want to do	0	1	2	3	4
54. I have to limit my social activity because I am tired	0	1	2	3	4

55. Looking at the above 20 questions, how much would you say these additional concerns affect your quality of life? (circle one)

1 2 3 4 5 6 7 8 9 10

Renal Preservation Diet

Renal Diet

Diet order

Calories: Adequate to achieve and maintain appropriate weight

Protein: 0.6 to 0.8 g/kg (60% high biologic value)

Sodium: 60 to 100 mEq (1.4 to 2.3 g) or as needed to limit fluid retention

Consult dietitian

Description

- Dairy products may be limited.
- Very small amounts of meat, limited amounts of breads and starches. Fruits and vegetables are allowed with the renal diet.
- Special low-protein products (low-protein bread and cookies), protein free modules (glucose polymers), and high calorie low protein foods (certain desserts, sweets, and fats) may be used to increase calorie intake.
- Table salt and commercially salted foods are excluded. Most foods should be prepared without adding salt.

Nutrient Value

- May not meet RDAs for protein
- Does not meet the RDAs for many vitamins and minerals, including calcium.

Comments

- Recommend a renal multivitamin and calcium supplement. Be cautious of supplements that contain phosphorus, potassium, magnesium, and vitamins A and D.
- Although hyperlipidemia and/or hypercholesterolemia may be present, dietary limitations of fat and cholesterol are not usually beneficial.
- Add dietary modifications for other medical problems to the diet order above.

Medical Nutritional Oral Supplements

(Nepro, Suplena)

Nepro contains increased levels of calcium, folic acid, pyridoxine and is low in sodium, potassium and phosphorus. It may be used as an oral supplement or as the primary source of nutrition for patients with acute or chronic renal failure who are receiving dialysis. Nepro may also be used in patients who are malnourished or are experiencing excessive proteinuria.

Suplena is low in magnesium, and vitamins A and D and has increased levels of calcium, folic acid, and pyridoxine. Suplena may be used as an oral supplement or as the primary source of nutrition for patients who are not receiving dialysis. In certain situations, Suplena may also be used by patients undergoing dialysis who need high calorie, low-protein supplement.

Low sodium diet

- Do not use salt at the table
- Use only half the amount of salt (or less) normally used in recipes and in cooking
- Learn to read food labels
- Avoid foods high in sodium, as listed below.

  - All salted or smoked meat or fish (bacon, Canadian bacon, corned beef, frankfurters/hot dogs, sardines, ham, herring, smoked fish, luncheon meats, smoked sausage, bratwurst, canned tuna, canned meat entrees)

  - Cheeses (camembert, cheese spreads, roquefort, gorganzola, processed cheese [Velveeta, American], party dips)

  - Breads and rolls with salt toppings

  - Convenience and processed foods (frozen dinners, oriental foods, spaghetti [commercial], pot pies, packaged entrees; rice, potato, and noodle mixes; potato chips, pretzels, salted nuts, crackers or popcorn, sauerkraut, tomato juice, canned tomatoes, sauce, and paste; bouillon cubes, gravy and sauce mixes; pickles, olives, relish; soups: canned, frozen, or dehydrated)

  - Seasonings that contain sodium (celery salt, chili sauce, garlic salt, lemon pepper, horseradish, onion salt, soy sauce, Lite salt, meat sauces, meat tenderizers, monosodium glutamate [MSG], seasoned salt, Worchestershire sauce, barbeque sauce)

  - Certain foods and condiments that are high in sodium should be used in moderation (peanut butter, catsup, commercial salad dressings)

Herb Chart

This list is a sampling of herbs commonly purported to aid in the following:

Asthma attacks	Caffeine, chili pepper, garlic, onion, horseradish, mustard
Blood clots	Onion, garlic, ginger, melon, kelp
Bronchitis/emphysema	Chili pepper, garlic, onion, mustard, horseradish, milk
Bronchitis and sinusitis	Various oil combinations of pine, thyme, lavender, mint, eucalyptus
Cancer	Broccoli, cabbage family, apple (possible), citrus fruits (possible), garlic (possible), licorice, soybeans
Caries	Tea, grape juice, black cherry juice, coffee, milk, cheese
Cholesterol (high level)	Oat bran, oatmeal, dried beans, soybeans, grapefruit segments and membrane, cumin, cinnamon, ginger, mustard, flaxseed, banana, plantain, apple
Colds and flu	Echinacea, chili pepper (decongestant), eucalyptus (decongestant)
Constipation	Cascara buckthorn, aloe, castor oil plant
Diarrhea	Apple juice, yogurt with live cultures, blackberries, black currants, honey
Headaches	Chili pepper, feverfew. Volatile oils release aromas from some plant flowers, leaves, and fruits; may produce mild stimulation, induce relaxation or aid in pain relief
Infection	Licorice, chamomile, garlic, onion, yogurt, apple, orange juice, tea, grape juice, blueberries, cranberries, peaches, figs
Insomnia	Hops, sugar, honey
Motion sickness	Ginger
Osteoporosis	Milk
Stroke	Fresh fruits, fresh vegetables, brown seaweed, black currants, blueberries
Throbbing pain	Chili pepper
Tumor growth	Certain ocean sponges, licorice, flaxseed
Ulcers	Umbelliferous vegetables (parsley, celery), banana, plants in cabbage family
Urinary tract infection	Cranberries, cranberry juice

Yakima Fruite Paste Recipe

DOSE: 1-2 tablespoons per day

> 1 pound prunes
> 1 pound raisins-pitted
> 1 pound figs
> 4 oz senna tea
> 1 cup brown sugar
> 1 cup lemon juice

1. Prepare tea-use about 2 1/2 cups boiled water added to tea and steep 5 minutes
2. Strain tea to remove tea leaves and add only 1 pint tea to a large pot, then add fruit.
3. Boil fruit and tea for 5 minutes.
4. Remove from heat and add sugar & lemon juice. Allow to cool.
5. Use hand mixer or food processor to turn fruit mixture into smooth paste.
6. Place in plastic container and place in freezer. (Paste will not freeze but will keep forever in freezer).
7. Spoon out what you require each day.

Enjoy eating fruit paste straight off the spoon.

Spread it on toast or add hot water and make a drink.

- If the fruit paste is not working (no bowel movements) then increase the amount of fruit paste each day)
- If the fruit paste induces very loose stools, cut down on the amount of fruit paste intake. Consider taking it every other day in some cases.
- For questions or problems with the fruit paste, contact your home care or hospice nurse.